DANCING WITH DEMENTIA

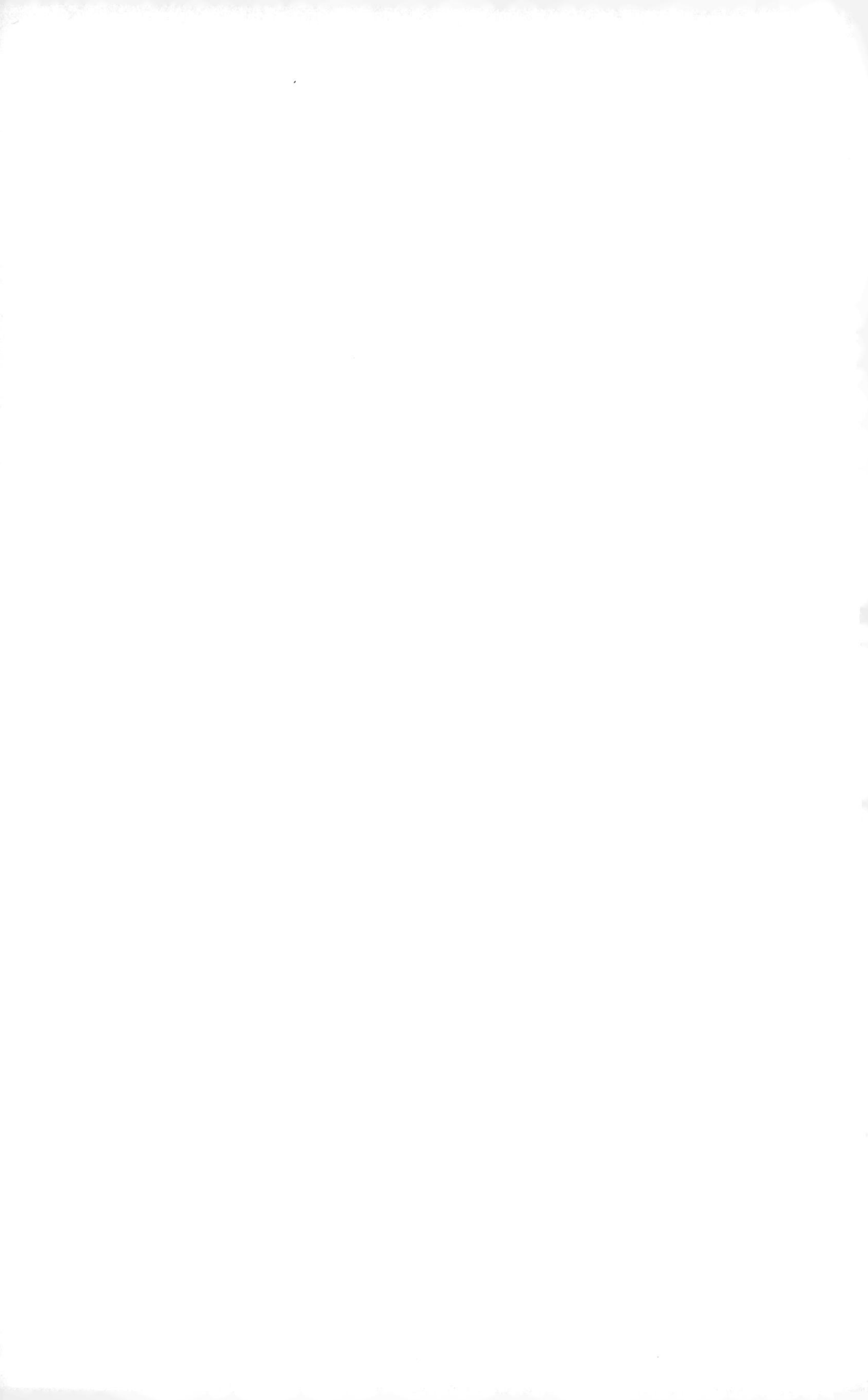

DANCING WITH DEMENTIA

Using the Art of Poetry to Become a Reflective Practitioner

Robert John Raingruber and

Bonnie Jean Raingruber

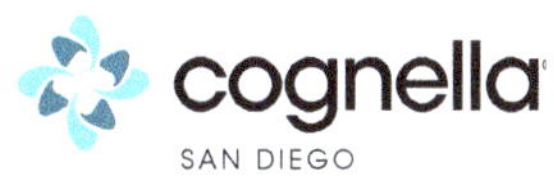

Printed in the United States of America.

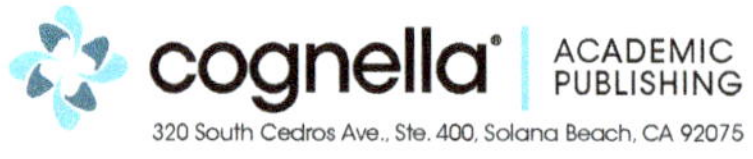

To Bright Dancer with all my love for Time and Eternity.

Brief Contents

Detailed Contents

Introduction

Reading and writing poetry are reflective practices. Reading and writing poetry helps a nurse thoughtfully attend to emotions that color practice, discover why particular clinical situations remain in awareness, develop insight into feelings, remember how patients and families feel, rethink solutions to clinical problems, as well as let go of intense clinical experiences. Reading and writing poetry are excellent ways to improve one's nursing practice.

This collection of poems was written by Robert Raingruber, a mathematician, teacher, poet, songwriter, athlete, and chess master as he had first begun his dissent into Lewy body dementia. Robert had an IQ of 140, loved words, spoke five languages, read the dictionary for fun, created 350 themed crossword puzzles, and wrote multiple songs. At the end of his journey tears fell down his cheek when words finally left him. These poems use the language of poetry, analogy, and metaphor to catalogue what it feels like to defy the developing dark, to know the chilling fear, dread, loss of control, loss of cherished memories, sadness, and enduring strength and comfort that are all a part of the journey of Alzheimer's and dementia. The collection ends with poems written by Bonnie, Robert's wife, a mental health clinical nurse specialist, as she walked with him. Writing was for her a way of coping and healing from the loss of her soul mate.

Included at the end of the book is a tutorial on how to develop your own poems, to journal and process the intense feelings and experiences that accompany working with families going through Alzheimer's and dementia. There are reflective practice questions designed to help you gain insight about yourself and your patients as well as develop professional expertise.

Schon (1983) emphasized that reflective practice is an important tool for improving one's nursing practice. Reflective practice is a habit of mind. It involves looking inward and examining our own responses as well as looking outward and carefully attending to the context of particular clinical situations (Kemmis, 1985). Reflective practitioners examine their beliefs, actions, and feelings in order to reframe situations, remain open to creative possibilities, align beliefs and actions, and develop expertise. Loughran (2002) emphasized that reflection is effective when "the practitioner comes to see and understand the practice setting from a variety of viewpoints" (p. 36). Reflection is a self-corrective process. By reflecting on past clinical situations and reconstructing the inherent possibilities, it is possible to adapt more quickly to future clinical challenges.

Within the reflective practice literature reflection and action are tied (Dewey, 1910). In this workbook, reading, reflecting, and completing exercises to promote writing about practice are emphasized. It is often in the action, in the writing about practice, that one comes to understand. Wheelock (1963) explained that "if a poet is troubled about an awareness, [they are] impelled to create a poem to embody the elusive preoccupation and reveal it to [them]self and others" (p. 31). Writing amplifies otherwise silent perceptions and impressions.

Nursing is an intense and challenging profession. Images from clinical practice "take root in us" and prompt us to notice emotional resonances that echo portions of our own life experience (Bachelard, 1969, p. xix). By writing poetry we are able to discover subtle details about our own values. Poets frequently complete a poem before discovering what it is about because only during the writing is the theme is fully developed. By writing we are able to reorganize and make something whole from feelings of pain and confusion (Wylie & Simon, 2002). A troubling, unresolved clinical situation is transformed into a product of value.

Poetry helps one develop "a gut level understanding of the meaning of things" (Gendlin, 1962, p. 11). Crawford (1993) stated that in nursing and in poetry we must see life bare and examine reality from a front row seat. In poetry and in nursing it is important to listen to the impressions we encounter, reflect on their personally felt significance, find an inner anchor or referent for the lingering impressions, and understand their implicit meanings. We need to examine the personal coloring we give to clinical situations and explore why we respond as we do.

Poetry develops within us "an increased capacity to provide compassionate care to those in need" (Connelly, 1999, p. 423). Poetry enhances one's capacity to understand oneself and other people. It permits us to develop our practice by reflecting on and sharing glimpses of others' life experience. Poetry provides "a time for reflection, a time to hear another's experience, a time for replenishment, a time for self-growth" (Friedrich, 1999, p. 1160).

Poetry helps us reflect on and value what is most important within life and within the nursing profession (Linney, 2000). "In its portrait and in its permanence, poetry refuses to let experiences, feelings, and images remain inconsequential, mundane, or insignificant" (Holmes & Gregory, 1998, p. 1194). Poetry is evocative by nature. It allows us to set aside everyday concerns and focus on significant experiences from our practice. Because being engaged in a situation is an antidote to burnout (Benner & Wrubel, 1989), poetry also helps to keep our love of nursing alive. Make time in your busy day to use some of the reflective practice questions at the end of this book and explore the helpful hints for writing poetry to develop your practice. Enjoy your journey.

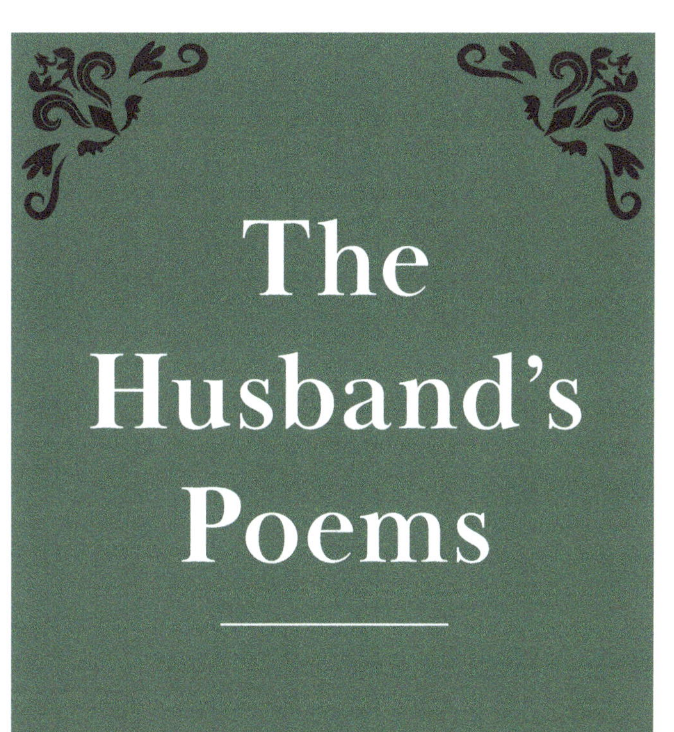
The
Husband's
Poems

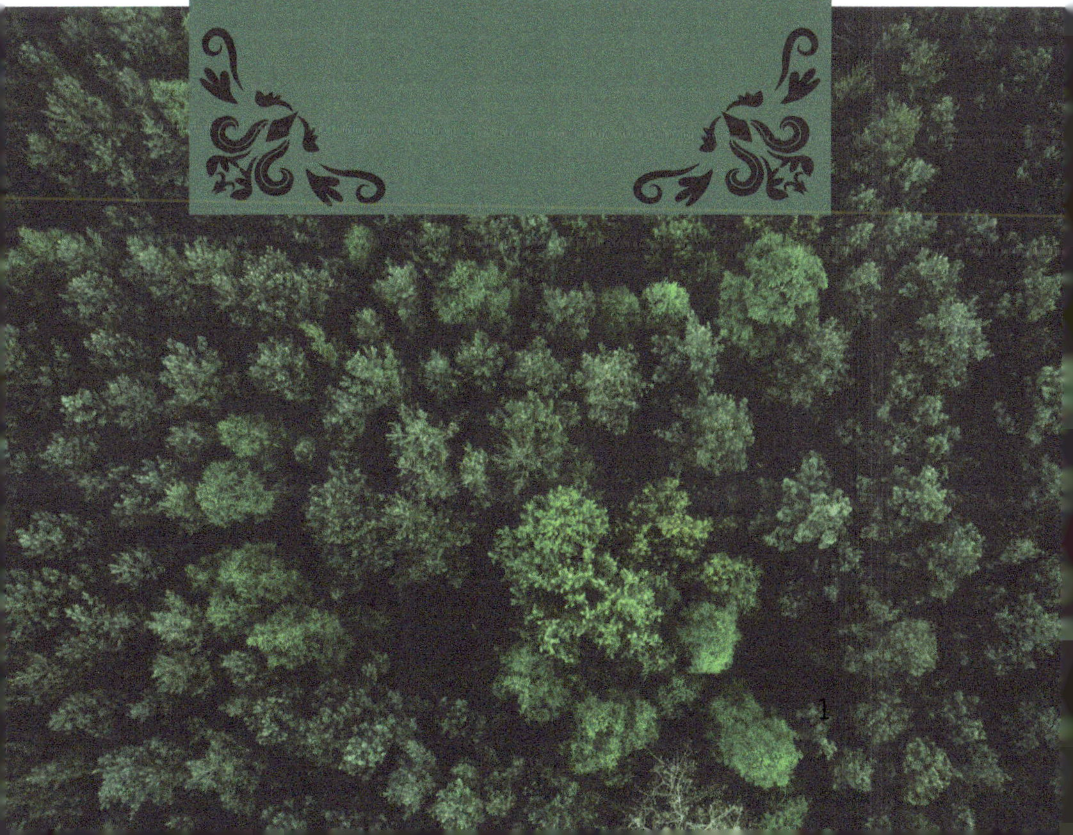

Fire on the Mountain

Just there a fire on the mountain saw I
In the distance beyond the great valley floor,
Conflagration untamed as it lingered ablaze,
And stood I transfixed when it captured my gaze—
Could it flout the dark waters of heavenly sky?

Not so I averred noting horizon's domain,
Being deftly encroached as I craved to see more,
Then finally quashed by the onrushing sea,
Eventide conquest of fire and me,
Left alone to digest what I could not contain.

With the hope of rekindling a flame or a spark
I looked toward the peak, blackened funeral pyre,
As pixie dust stars tickled fancy-less night
And stillness resided in lieu of the light.
When the fire on the mountain was vanquished by dark.

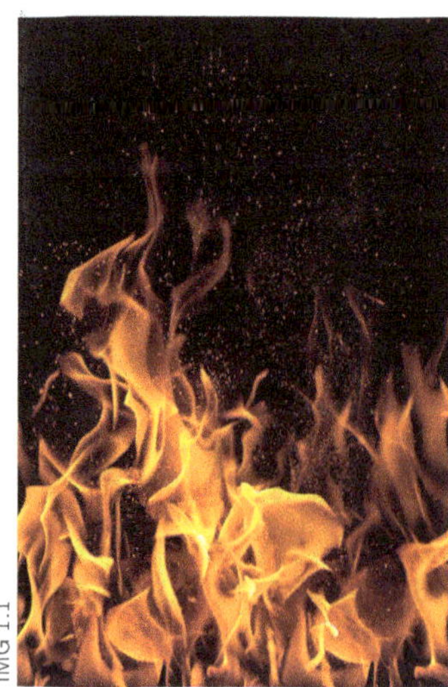
IMG 1.1

Apostrophe to Dark

O Dark, you like Venetian shades are drawn,
Your swarthy cloak enwrapping pallid night;
Mysterious, your murky palms enshroud
The neon light arenas of the town.

O Dark, the eerie peal of church bells sets
Upon the heart and renders it afraid,
And dulled convolutions slow respond
To messages on windows, walls, and doors.

O Dark, the void is bleakly met
In the enigma of reality,
As dead marquees stir recollections dim
Of pictures, massive screens, and velvet seats.

O Dark, your silence feels like falling leaves
Entrenching me in covert reverie,
Alone to walk in dread of glow-less lamps
While seeking places where long shadows are.

Yet even as you veil me now, O Dark,
Up past a steeple tower un-needing prayers
I go secure, my soulless predator,
That somewhere in this black a light is warm.

Sapphire Sun

Sodden sun buttering pale autumn sky
Hot dry air still, like the water below
Scrub jay objecting to afternoon balm
Hawk overheard like a kite on the high.

A single gray cloud near horizon doth lie
In wait for the golden God journeying calm
Reflecting on shimmering downriver flow
It cradles proud sun now a sapphire blue eye.

Witness a leaf untethered waft light
Breeze battered downstream where rock ripples go
Beneath menacing clouds whose black puffs billow free
At last raging round fire is nowhere in sight.

Relentless this river, from trickle to stream
Quickens to falls on the way to the sea
And cat paws become pelting storm in the night
As dark blankets all in an unending dream.

Shadows of the Night

Shadows of the day I see,
Sights along a trodden shore,
A long trek on a redwood's trail,
A picnic in some lonely park,
Flashing on sun days of yore.

Downtown café lunch at noon,
Fish harbor seagulls screeing loud,
April flowers in desert veil,
Alpine slopes white canopy,
And any place to lose the crowd.

But what, you ask, when coming dark
Overrides the sounds that bent the ears,
Of round promises by summer moon,
Vain carnival of sights and smells,
Which only signaled urgent fears.

Sundown painted sky impels
Today, as dark overtakes the light,
My storied eyes in love with her—
Though shadows of the day are gone,
Not so the shadows of the night.

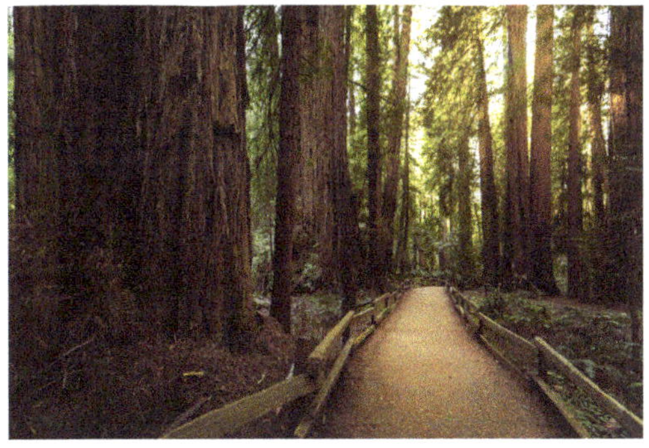

IMG 1.2

Fire

Fire dances, fire sings
    Crackled paeans, ochred wings
        Flames a-licking unseen things

Fire hisses, fire heaves
    Spitted embers, searing sheaves
        Blaze a-torching learning leaves

Fire fiddles, fires scores
    Ardent tunes, ancient lores
        Hearth a-glowing idea stores

Fire gorges, fires stakes
    Frenzied fevered log which bakes
        Spark a-yearning, heart with ache

Fire dances, fire sings
    Crackled paeans, ochred wings
        Flames a-licking unseen things.

IMG 1.3

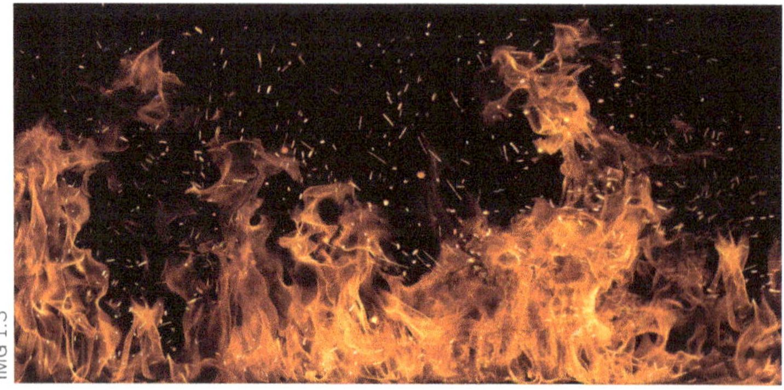

Coves

I put canoe out on the water
And awkward did I oar the drift:
Lithe bending dell stream jostled me—
I lost control it was so swift—
I wide of eye from things to see.

Branch overhang to duck beneath,
Thick snag ahead to bypass low,
Near widened river sandbar bend,
And so pacific was the flow
That it seemed not to have an end.

I bye the bye espied a cove
And followed close the shore inside
To find a cat-tailed universe
Where mallards mingled, and swans would glide
And butterflies their dance rehearse.

I, soon to wend my way downstream,
And in seeming endless coves,
Did rachet up my leisured pace,
Where sundry hazards lurked in droves,
Fear first made manifest on my face.

Then as I fought to ply my oar
Against foes currents, I understood
The vainness of my hope to slow
My seaward surge; as well I could,
I savored coves I'd come to know.

A Fruitless Chinese Pistachio Fall

Fruitless Chinese pistachio trees
Line both sides of narrow Wellesley Lane,
A winding dark-green tunnel, vail legacy
Of torpid waning summer.

November leaves, bestirred by autumn's chill,
Almost overnight rebel en masse, bedaubed with
A mater's strokes of amber hues and crimson,
A cacophony of stain.

A rustling breeze arouses these time pages
From smold'ring slumber, whence winter's breathy blasé
Unleashes sparks, creating in its wake
An aborning holocaust.

A fortnight fails to quell the raging flame;
But slow December, not so far behind,
Finds stain and burning purged, proud leaves bestrewn
Like yesterday's newspaper.

The furies of dead January's storms—
Ice and rain—assault beleaguered earth,
Its trees, belying distant cycling rumblings
Of canvas oils and fire.

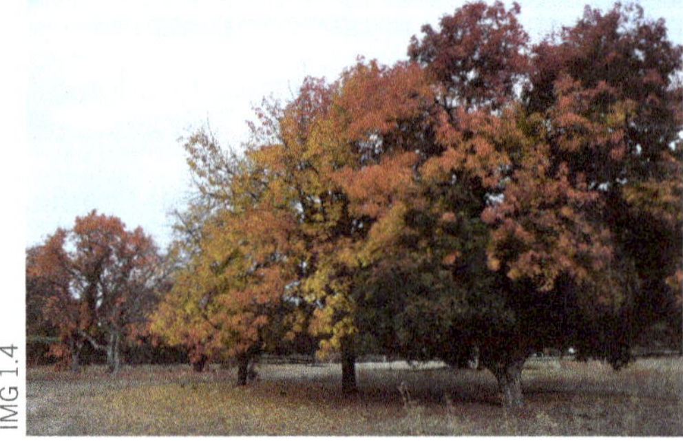

IMG 1.4

Horseshoe Bend

Viewed from a lawn chair on a weathered deck pier
At backyard's end, a tiny swirl of water
Sprightly pirouettes like a whirling arms-in ballerina.
Here an azure swatch of a transferred sky,
There shimmering eggshell licks, small blinds
Endlessly opening and closing.

Before, the water is khaki green, faithfully
Reflecting thick foliage from opposite bank,
Shrub and blackberry lined, with great river oaks
Vying with locust trees and tall cottonwoods
Stretching obliquely over the water for some space,
So close that they feel within reach.

In the stand of trees there a branch cracks, breaking up
A resonant calm, and lands with a thud. A red-tailed
Hawk, circling high beyond, seeks out a pasture meal,
While a swooping blackbird is a mere ebon blur
Just above the waterline. The wayfaring winds
Tree-hisses become engulfed by rhythmic clicks

Of a laden freight train roaring over a trestle
Above a lush riverbend bank of wild grapevines
Dusk approaches. Almost in unison are heard the distinctive
Caws of an unseen crow, only now drowned out by the shrill
Whistle of the train. For a few moments a river moth
And falling leaf in flight appear to dance together.

The soft plook of a fish is heard and ripples follow
Ever widening. Beavers poke their heads up
Downstream as the color of the river begins to
Change accommodating the dying sun. There is
A chill this June eve here at the horseshoe bend
Of the Mokelumne river where life eddies.

The Kite

White ghosting sun in a wispy cloud
Which blustering winds of March assail
A stripling boy charged wildly by
Upwind. His hands upraised unveil

A weathered string unwinding slow
And stretching taut to wing'ed kite.
When suddenly it lurched up high
Climbing till near lost to sight.

Still vagabonding to and fro,
All but lifting lad off trail,
This tussling wind and wing uncowed,
The kite broke free. Some say the gale,

Some say the boy, but if I might,
The kite it was that willed the flight.

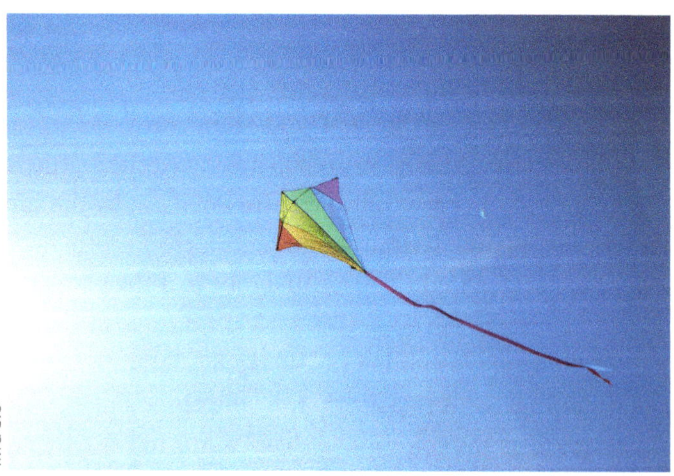
IMG 1.5

Robert Raingruber, "The Kite" from "Hourglass and Nine Other Poems," Qualitative Inquiry, vol. 12, no. 4, pp. 752.

November Leaf

November leaf all yellowed and browned
Did fall from a tree and drift to the ground.
Said leaf green and bright and a-billowing once
On a branch of rich insignificance
Makes way for spring buds when winter is spent;
We are in no wise entitled to misrepresent
All value ascribed to this sheaf that I see—
However, we like it are part of the tree.

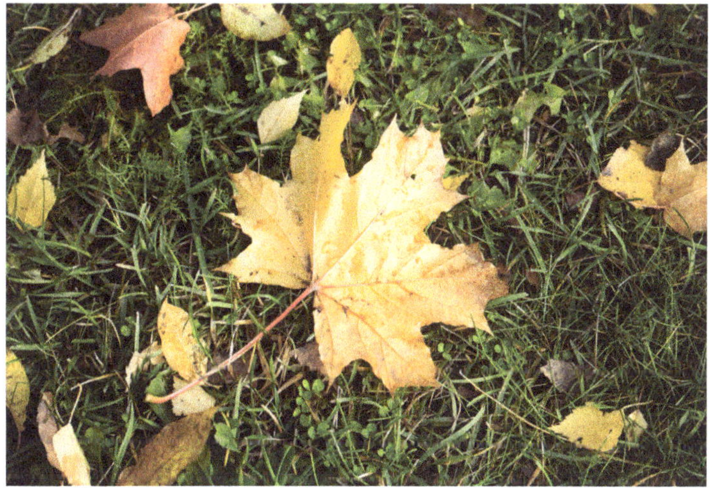

IMG 1.6

Red Embering Skies

Alone am I walking midst saguaro and sage,
Joshua trees here providing no shade,
Autumn's bright sun in fine grandeur displayed,
Seeming to float this October parade.

Desert breeze stirs desolation expanse,
Sand twisters awhirl in chase of themselves
While the great plodding ball among caressing pastels
Goes impacting horizons the deeper it delves.

Worn sun gasping now in a fiery rage
Wreaks a havoc of hues assaulting my eyes,
Through knowing its destiny, it vainly defies
So that all that remains lie red embering skies.

Who stands to track barren flaming of life,
Of flashing and flaring, pursing some mark,
And what of the chasing with vigor and spark,
Awhirl to protest the developing dark?

Cloud Shadows

Near the top of the mountain, I had settled upon
As nighttime departed, came cresting at dawn
Majestic magenta then rich hues of red
On thin patchworks of clouds hung loosely ahead.

Just below them appearing on rocks, shrubs and trees,
Fleece shadows-and they-now heeding a breeze
As yawning sun neared the late of the day
Clouds and cloud shadows did wither away.

I admit I did hark to the considerable sight
Of the cottony tufts and their shadowing plight-
Are we not clouds in suspension arrayed?
Whereby memoried shadows will echo our fade?

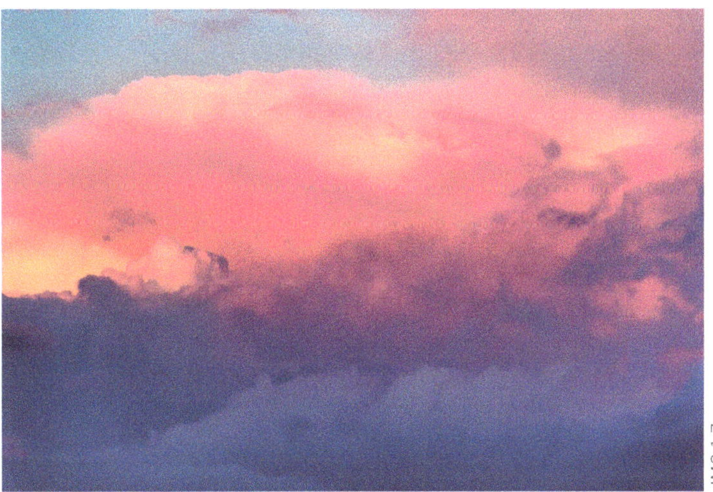

IMG 1.7

Diamonds on the Water

Whither blowest locust tree breeze
Stirring lacy leaves aflutter
Midst baking summer arcing sun
Causing flowing stream to sputter

All in a moment there they shimmered
Sparkling proud, a blinding whit
Some thousand diamonds on the water
Reflections of ephemeral light

Flushed with stirring memories
Through fractal lenses brief I see
Precious scenes, a shining love
Arresting time once took from me

Whither goest waning sun
Veiled reminder of Beauty's daughter
I know I'm cursed to dwell again
Upon the diamonds on the water.

The Dragon

The dragon breathed a fork'ed fire
On huddled clouds in sky forlorn
Affrighting lost vacating dark
And signaling first blush of morn.

Harkened I to caucused crows
Berating hushed benighted dream
As scurrying squirrels thrifted nuts
Near sandbar beach by slothful stream.

Wondered I in awe and dread
Whence came this dragon in the night
Fending off November's chill
And putting torch to all in sight.

Where went the beastly warming glow
When sparrow chorus filled the day,
All silenced by a soundless roar
Ere the dragon slinked away.

So, daylight deed becomes a dream,
When chastened I by dark and death,
Returning night might spell the spark
But not extinguish dragon's breath.

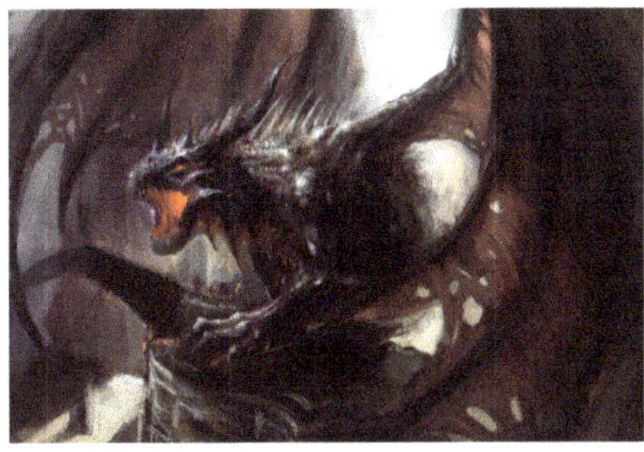

IMG 1.8

Dream

I looked out on the water
It seemed to me like glass
No wind-whips marred its surface
No ripple from a bass
A weighty stillness sitting
Dusk mirror come to pass

I closed my eyes and listened
But strange there was no sound
From frogs on water lilies
Or crickets on the ground
No cries from wing'ed shorebirds
Or willow whispers to be found

No ships sailed on the water
No men with nets ashore
Or footsteps in the beach sand
No children to adore
Nor forest huts or pathways
Or laughter, love and more.

Then I found myself awaken
Red dawn-light crowding dark
Whitecaps laced the sea as
Hissing breezes left their mark
And palms on shore were swaying

Gloried sun peeked out from
Horizon's line it gleamed
Foaming Earth around me living
Made an empty death it seemed
Now Nature joins me jeering
The nightmare I had dreamed.

Flamingo Sky

O flamingo sky again
You flaunt to me your hark'ning hues,
Fleece everglades of pinks and jades
Which dying sun imbues.

Haste, away, flamingo sky,
And yield to tardy darkness tease;
End reveried thought your presence wrought
And mend my heart unease.

Cloud tufts return you, flamingo love,
Sweet flesh so fragile, rose and wan,
In florid times and clovered climes,
My jewel of yore is gone.

Mendocino

North, on the California coastline through oak-pocked hills,
Whose Thornbush sprays and Manzanita outline
Aged leaning cabins midst browned waving grasses,
With a dying embered sun in a losing joust with murky, nimbus sky
I drive. Highway 1 twisting along the edge of precipices
Which tumble down into shadowed canyons.
Just then, around a bend through a vagrant stand of pines,
Eerily ablaze with golden streams of dusk light
Appears Mendocino, a lacy frill of clapboard houses
On a bluff, and white cottages, and charming inns
Whose restaurant walls depict much headier logging days
Of this Victorian headland port town in a bygone era.
Stubborn townfolk and free-spirited, slow recast as an artist colony,
And still regarding strangers with a raised brow, beckon
Watchers to the seaboard cliffs, outbraving whale-hunters.
Suddenly about this village pearl, shrouded by cold Pacific waters
And pristine interior redwood forest, lightning puts the
Saw to darkened sky, yielding in its wake to companion thunder.
Windshield droplet cat paws give way to steady pelting drops,
And for a moment a blustering mindless wind swoops over land
To seascape, framing unstitched time. At town's end parked
Where fathomless universe is sea-edged, as darkness envelops
The spraying heavens. I close my eyes in league with tranquil
Earth, harkening to the soft sweet ditty of the rain.

Patterns

By dark behold the Universe without,
Which, replicating a mosaic one year past,
Does serve us notice of a future night
To think about.

Beyond the purview of our ears and eyes
No less a problem is the microcosm
Of atoms, which confirm more laws eternal
For us to prize.

Garden Earth, we look to you for lines
Of symmetries in bulbs and honeycombs,
While crystal flakes of snow and rainbows arced
Bestow designs.

The world we live bespeaks defining themes
Redundant, such as baseball and chess;
Our mind—our soul—must it be as unique
As changing dreams?

Nay. We stand too close to recognize the paradigm,
For change is just a higher plane example—
It is our senses that betray us through
Opaque-windowed time.

We do what we have but already done.
We learn again past thought already known,
It is the future that we see—life patterns
And we are one.

River's Edge

Mid dropping sunlight feath'ring gold
On gentle flowing river's mane
I saw again your dancing eyes
Impelled by siren seaward swain.

As swallows rock on Greenleaf Willows
An oak ball glides without a sound,
Near river's edge this swirling dervish,
But ne'er to root on solid ground.

Where went the time from flake to falls
O meandering soulless pearl
That wings me round, a lover's haunting,
Like an oak ball in a whirl.

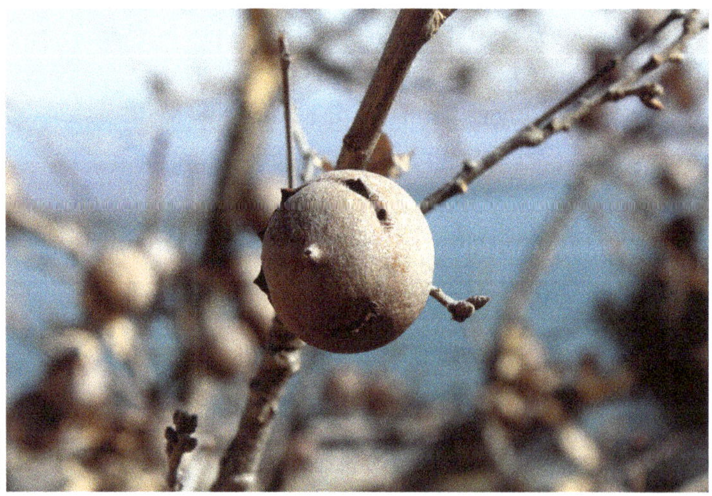
IMG 1.9

Ripples

A dogwood
tree overhangs a glassy pond. It's ocher
autumn leaves glisten, mirroring
the light from fading day
At twilight, a
cricket fiddles while
the sky burns, a laden quiet
overcomes the pool and its environs.
All at once a soldier leaf makes war on the
viscous water plane, creating a
ripple. Then another
leaf enlists
forming ever-widening
circles in sycophantic imitation.
The violated pond, approaching calm,
appears dusky as the dying sky, its ripples
having declared their freedom, decamp, and the water
transmutes to darkened crystal. Now only Venus
is reflected on its surface. Introspectively,
awaiting another invader leaf, she
wonders whether the next
ripple has a chance
to last.

Felicitous Dawn

We determined to take a walk in the park—
A journey we ventured other times in the dark,
And where we had kindled the very first spark.

Two benches did beckon, we lingered behooved
To talk of the very path we had grooved
While far constellations silently moved.

Familiar it felt, but in the shadows, we knew...
Something amiss between me and you.
Thus lay our chance, had we mending to do?

Mountain and sea, sea and sand in the flow—
How had it been, when did it show,
What had it meant, and where did it go?

As we both reckoned the course we were on,
Horizon hues reddened, and the truth was foregone;
We took our own leave of felicitous dawn.

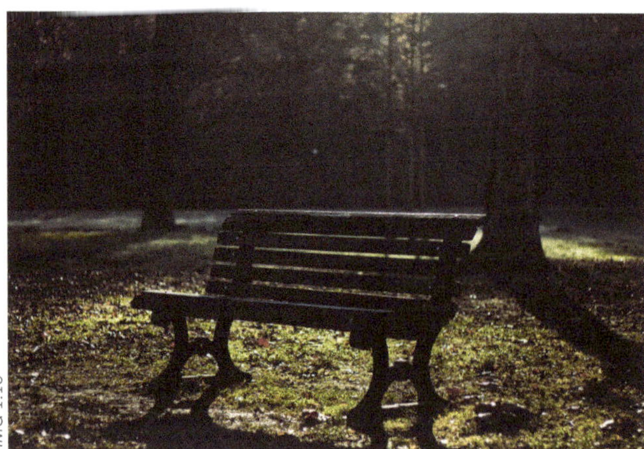

IMG 1.10

Turning a Page

Great tomes on the shelves
Paginated and bond
And hinting good use
By their spine can be found.

Old smell of such works
In a library refined
Is certainly a lure
Of an elegant kind.

But heightened emotion
As the senses engage
Only really occurs
When turning a page.

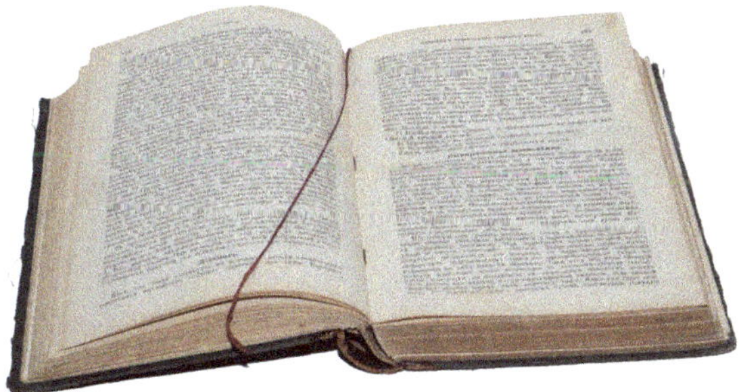

IMG 1.11

Why Hangs a Shroud

Why hangs a shroud o'er the saber of Truth
When behold 'tis emblazoned and starkly arrayed,
Ours to indulge and immerse in our youth,
Yet often mishandled at twists of its blade—
Is it forsooth but the way we were made?

And why hangs a shroud o'er the essence of Life,
Perceives as our destiny much as our right;
Why should there be one iota of strife
Entangling our thoughts and so blurring our sight,
A circumstance rife with bemusing delight?

Why hangs a shroud o'er the bright lamp of Love
Which emanates warmth midst a radiant glow—
Enchanted by such iridescence above
We envelop ourselves satisfied that we show
Quite enough of heart-world wonders in toe.

Sandy Albums

Albums filling counters, halls,
Divert the heart and mind and eyes
With hopeful times and places seen,
Enriched by family ties.

Albums, captured hearth and home,
Your bricks and boards and yard rejoiced
At each sound of laughter heard
And infant's cry of pain there voiced.

Albums, in one blink of eye,
Snapshots pressed on page and wall
A hurricane did wipe away,
Evidence of it all.

Life

Life is like a book
With a beginning and an end,
The pages in between
Be careful not to bend.

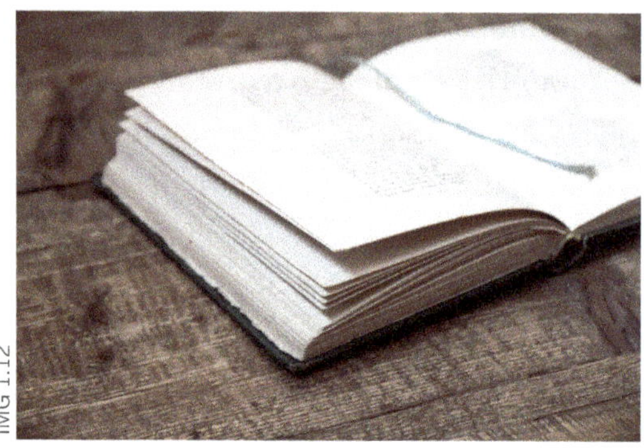

IMG 1.12

Storm

Behold yon rolling, retching sky;
Its baleful billows, staining dark,
As nerves of light electrify
In blinding flashes stark,
Yield meek to mighty thunder's cry

Arrest these warlike peals and light
Lest rain and terrored wild beset
Benignant soil and sea with fright;
If only love fends off the went
Then all the world doth mend tonight.

Glaciers

Rivers of ice, long, long ago born
Inch their way forward majestic, forlorn
Till their arrival well after the wait.
Creaking and calving out into the strait.
Floes of ice glistening in peeks from the sun
Meander and bob melting until they are gone.
We are a glacier, generations of floes,
Glistening, meandering, and so it goes.

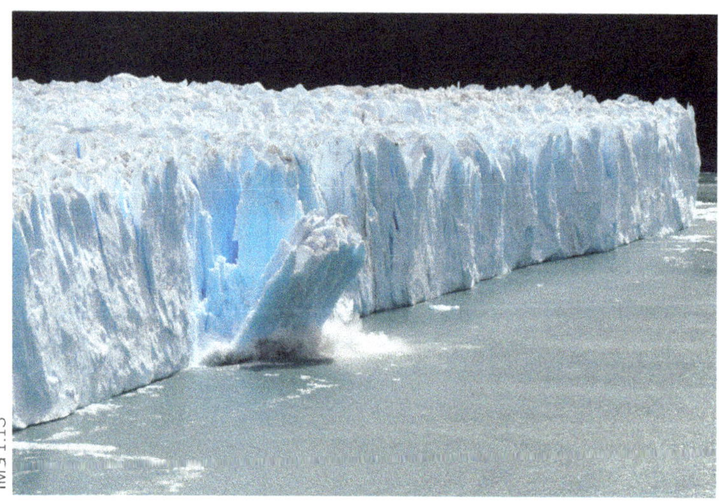

IMG 1.13

A Fire in the Sky

I saw a fire in the sky
A wild wind fanned the blaze
Violent voice to tortured craze
And left alone to ache and cry
I saw a fire in the sky.

I felt her storm in my veins
Which mulling mind could not mend
A pounding pouring without end
And though I raged against the rains
Remained the storm in my veins.

She surged electric in my soul
Spearing spasms reaching deep
Mid silent screams in my sleep
I sensed her bolting rays control
And surge electric in my soul.

I saw a fire in the sky
Which dousing dark could not quell
From the ether to the hell
And I winced and wondered why
There was a fire in the sky.

The Light

Dark-shine,
Black space intruder,
Scenting out cranny defilements
In pitchy forest primeval
And deep mountain mine.

Linger, eyes
Sight organ sensors,
On night's ill-begotten behaviors
Around inky chasms oceanic
And distant jet skies.

Rampage on,
Eviling darkness,
Persisting in caging bright energy—
Delusion of grandeur fantastic—
In caverns far-gone.

Dare the glow
To refract or absorb,
Wishful of muting its radiance—
Its warmth—to blue earth's ebon canyons
And valleys below.

See the light,
Blazing unbound and benign,
Thou Sable Enemy, bearding
Blind ignorance and raven servitude,
Outlasting the night.

Dusk Berries

Raspberry hillcone melting away.
Blueberry pie line besting the day.
Gooseberry ripples in cloud lines play.

Strawberry soda spilling still.
Boysenberry wafers cooling the hill.
Blackberry sky tarts bake at will.

Raspberry hillcone turning maroon.
Blueberry, blackberry give way to moon.
Gooseberry, strawberry rise again soon.

Investiture

It is not with subtlety of pen
But with patent ring of cutlass steel
That markets, summ'ning hordes of panting men,
Are honed by competition midst lusty aims—
Betimes their siren calls are heard and heeded.

Unfettered minds invoke beguiling chance;
Blind strings of numbers stand like dandelions,
Whose out-stretched petals strut in random dance,
Chafed by willow rain and vagrant wind—
Unennobled goal more envied than exceeded.

A whimper rises to oppose the crash
Of tidal cymbals over shoreline rocks,
Defying business wisdom, while wagered cash
Stands conceived infertile—in its stead,
Investments made in world and people needed.

Floes of Ice

Great banks of ice lined the hillsides at dawn,
Glistening majestic and morning beguiled,
Their broken-off flows bobbing gently offshore
In a canyon whose river wound narrow and wild.

Buffeted lightly by a summery breeze
And tugged by a current flowing restive and free,
These floes of ice, busily harnessing sun,
Did take in the ride on the way to the sea.

The floes hit a rapids and, as thawing occurred,
The zenith of day became only a gleam;
The sea but siren did beckon them on
But all trace of the floes was gone from the stream.

Teutonic Idyll

In the Straits of Magellan blows frigid and raw
A squall gusty and violent, the dread williwaw.
    An old mill by marsh grasses, cattails, and reeds
    Near a pond in a valley is nestled sublime'
    Heaven's blue and fleece clouds, looking round you can see
    Dragonflies helicoptering past overgrown weeds
    And white swan flotillas of grace gliding by.
False doldrums reside, in a blink then are gone
Crisp broken by whitecaps appearing anon.
    Pond mirror is blackened by shadowy sky
    Offended by droplets which gloss to the lea
    A blinding ripsaw rent asunder the night
    Unleashing a torrent ne'er known from on high,
    Wreaking maximal havoc and fear in our time.
All the bowels of the earth open up to the wrath
As the williwaw rages unchecked in its path.
    Lea and pond are ablaze with cannons and fire
    Thunderous night claps reverberate so
    That returning dawn orb is a figment of light
    And yet the lea witnessed abating entire
    Firmament discord with the mill pond below.
Be wary of rock shoals, once pommeled perforce,
Lest an Aryan squall resume former course.

Igloo

Slightly curved blocks of fresh compacted snow
Lay scattered in masses on snow-whited tundra,
Where powdery flakes, like a flowing star-sky.
Swirled round and round a half-built arc'd home.

Defying November's untamed whistling winds,
A sled drawn by Eskimo dogs nigh approached;
Halting, an old light-brown man of flat face
And stocky build slow unloaded home blocks.

He revered childhood, hours spent with his father—
Artic skills, artisan from whalebone axes
To caribou clothes' his gone father's hand steeped
In this ice home facsimile, a reindeer day's walk

To the village; from there you could see the black waters,
Home to his boy ten sun-summers ago.
As winter day dimness succumbed to dead night,
On finishing he weary-viewed his strained work.

Sleep-conjuring Eskimo dreams of the spring-melt
Upcoming, enwrapping mist memories stored home
In his unconscious, his many sun-summers friend
And life partner since three dark days home floe departed.

The Name of Tomorrow

Burbling springs and playful rivulets
Converge in widening goose-necked streams,
Snaking slow and roaring, endlessly, on
Inexorable journeys to the sea.

An ebon speckled sky begins to yield to
Aborning light, anon to own the heavens
For some hours; external nightly rhythms
Decree the sky again decay to dark.
    And the name of today is tomorrow,
    And tomorrow has no name.

A mountain fusses, belching gas and rock,
Creating ceaseless black and fiery red
Lava rivers, ravenous as earthquakes
To achieve dominion of the land.
    And the name of today is tomorrow,
    And tomorrow has no name.

Perennial lightening sets pine needles, piled
Thick with forest birch leaves, smoldering,
Soon to be a wall of cageless fire,
Sometime silenced by a drenching storm.

Across nocturnal skies go shooting stars,
Unending fireworks which strafe galactic realms in
A hot celestial race to blackened earth,
To be buried in horizon's graveyard.
    And the name of today is tomorrow,
    And tomorrow has no name.

Love, a cosmic energy in powered
Fits and starts of timeless shade and light,
Flows, unremitting, uncontained—a mammoth
Tremored cauldron of furnace flame and fume.

Thunderbolts and holocausts demur,
While meteors abscond when Love is full;
At times chameleon, Love unceasing changes,
Making poignant noises, sputtering to nil.
    And the name of today is tomorrow,
    And tomorrow has no name.

I Thrilled at the Words

I thrilled at the words which sprang from page,
Which I eagerly read, now mellowed with age;
From the hearth were this raised nuanced lines aptly phrased,
Not stale as old cake, which is now all the rage.

It remained in my head long past did this verse,
A faceted gem not to lightly disburse
But to brandish and hold like a wineglass of old.
Or a potion, a brew, dispelling a curse.

Now weathered and worn and valued for naught.
Full up with crisp meaning its language had wrought,
It depicted a truth which spoke of vain youth.
And I thrilled at the words, bright canvas of thought.

From a time before words left me.

The Ultimate Traveler

Partaking of beauty of faraway places,
To tend to the cultures of alien store,
Imbibe of the waters of wide empty spaces
Impounding the energy needed to course
Through canyons and valleys to life's very source.
To stand in the shadow of obelisks distant
Or bask in the sun on a lonely ag'd shore;
To merit a love which seems nonexistent,
Enfolding the seed of all knowledge refined
Gives pause to the trav'ler who treks in his mind.

Hourglass

An irregular web on a tough silk
strand supporting a cotton-like sac of eggs
lies hidden in a dark nook under
a decaying woodpile. There
standing watch is
a shiny black
spider
whose globular
abdomen is bedaubed
with a rouge hourglass. She
appears serene, her soon-hatching
young safe from the lesser absent mate, a
venom victim, his time being up.

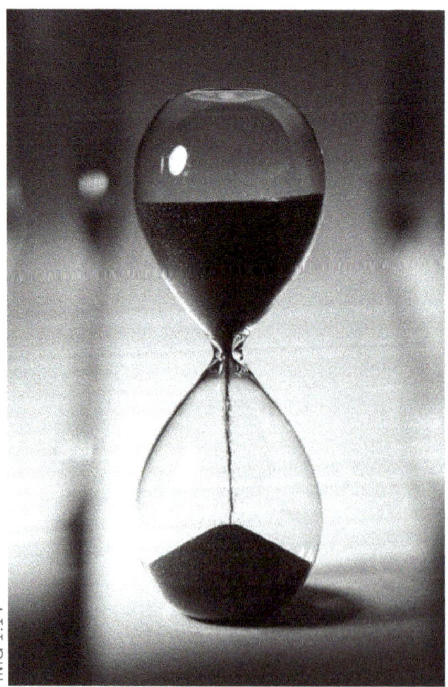
IMG 1.14

Credits

IMG 1.1: Copyright © 2010 Depositphotos/duskbabe.

IMG 1.2: Copyright © 2018 Depositphotos/mblach.

IMG 1.3: Copyright © 2017 Depositphotos/vero_ro39.

IMG 1.4: The Fun Chronicles, https://www.flickr.com/photos/196406308@N04/53334423089/in/photolist-8oxfQd-8UkbeN-8Uh8JP-8Uhf2H-2kV9ACY-5NEFkT-9BStxj-2iP7eB3-2iP9WPN-gG6rqy-gG6T3B-8eEtuu-2pfYigh-2pfYU56-8eBaQM-8eEvj7-2pfZsov-2pfSAN2-9BSjFn-2n9KPnB-2n9KPrK-2n9TWic-2n9Repk-2n9Re7S-2n9TWuK-2pfZsB6-2pfYRKG-2pfYRQM-2pfYRHx-2pfYRKm-2pfYihV, 2023.

IMG 1.5: Copyright © 2018 Depositphotos/Pakhnyushchyy.

IMG 1.6: Copyright © 2019 Depositphotos/ElenaNoeva.

IMG 1.7: Copyright © 2019 Depositphotos/fee76.

IMG 1.8: Copyright © 2012 Depositphotos/fotokostic.

IMG 1.9: Copyright © 2019 Depositphotos/hecos.

IMG 1.10: Copyright © 2021 Depositphotos/FabianoWaewell.

IMG 1.11: Copyright © 2013 Depositphotos/mercava2007.

IMG 1.12: Copyright © 2017 Depositphotos/azatvaleev.

IMG 1.13: Copyright © 2017 Depositphotos/durktalsma.

IMG 1.14: Copyright © 2021 Depositphotos/Fotofabrika.

The Wife's Poems

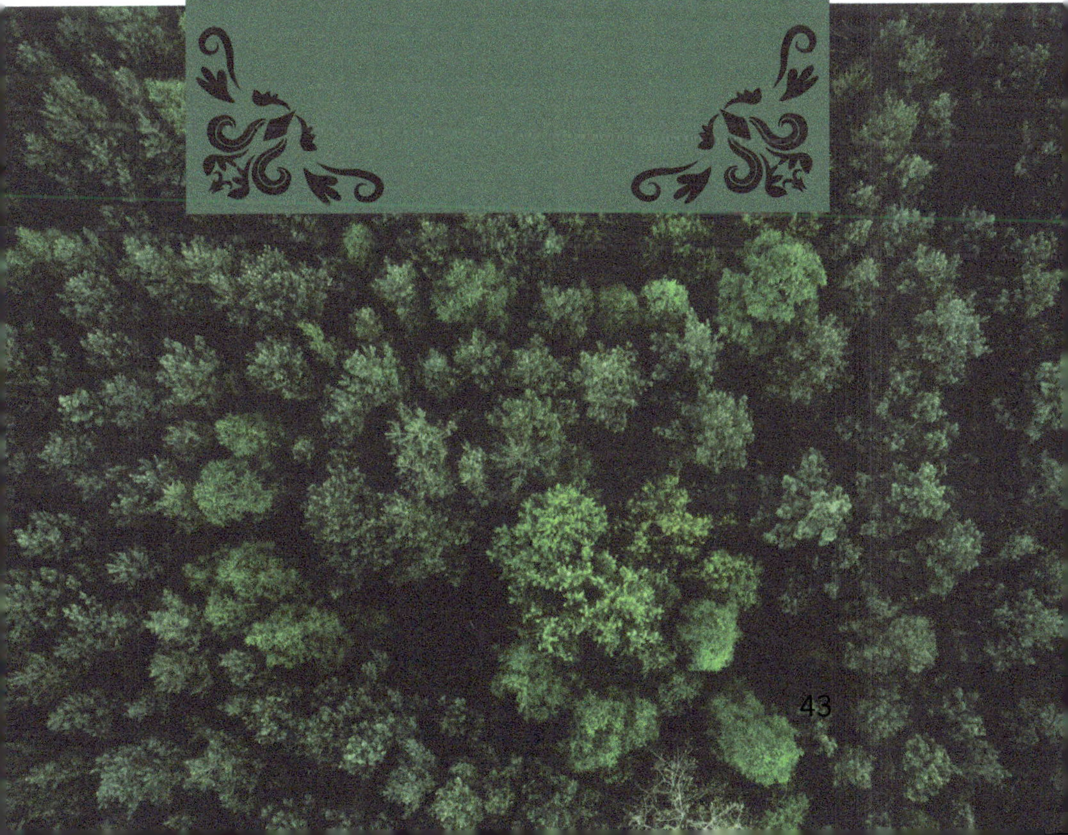

The Hawk

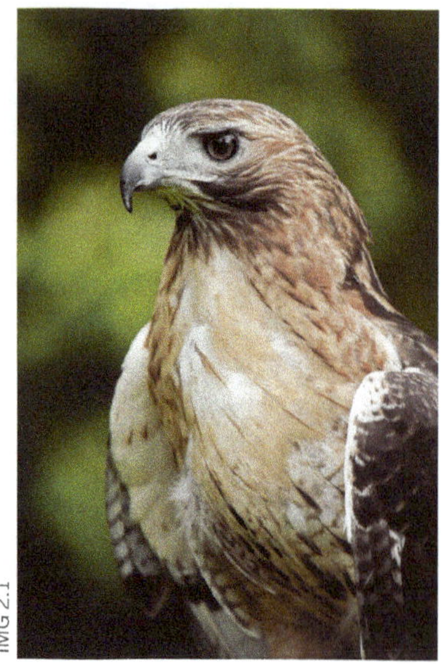
IMG 2.1

It is the winter of sadness
A hawk sits on dead branch
Searching for her mate.
The day is grey—foggy.
—The kind of a day
When you can't see into the future.

So, she huddled alone
In the cold twilight
Awaiting her blinking star.
The river below mirrored
No hope, no happiness this night.
She didn't know when

To move to a new perch
—A new perspective.
Where would this meandering
Stream of fate take her next?
She drew her black feathers in--
Shiny armor against the cold.

~~Gentle-Fluttered Partings~~

Dandelion bouquets
Cover the tombstone of
My husband, spreading still.

Blown too soon, we all are
White-petal-stripped,
Green stems standing

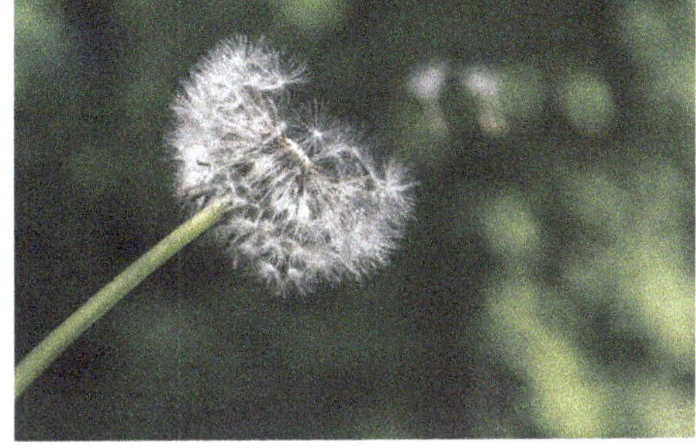
IMG 2.2

Bold upright and alone.
Tender seed carried and
Yet carries joy abroad

Landing soft, returning
Home, wrapped in gossamer
White, sprouting still.

Pain flutters, scattering
The wind—hushed
By butterfly wings.

Wishes reach out, waiting
Space to word, for his wisdom
Yet walks with silence, with calm.

Snow fluttering gentle
O'er my empty heart—memory
Visits—love outlasting life.

Pain Wilts Away

Persimmons bangle bright,
On leafless skeleton branch.

Winter wilts itself brittle and rose petals
Persist, hanging dry to the thorn.

Under a black and blue sun, the twig
Turns scarlet, separating itself from trunk.

Ice plant veins crack cold,
Taking us to blood-red aquifers.

Hawks circle above as breathless peace
Builds its strength and will not blow

Spanish moss to a darker olive hue. Lichen
Hair is suspended like the Time of Joys.

Same-shaded, ash-brown hills and trees lie
Invisible. Pampas grass feathers white with a fern.

Grapevined hillsides pincushion precisely.
Firewood fences weather irregular.

Confusion curds fractal
From this, a buttermilk sky.

Clouds Zorro the heavens, zippering into eternity
As dehiscent mortality awaits its opening.

Zigzag flutterings and migrations
Take twelve birds to the Holy Land.

As death approaches, inland rivers push the ocean out,
Traveling to the tip of the world on Hwy 1.

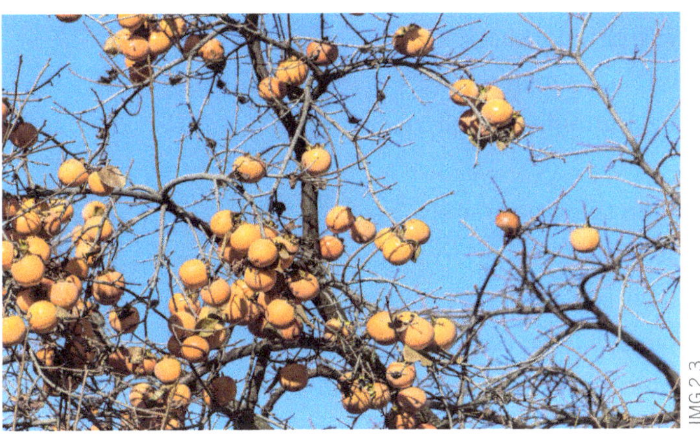
IMG 2.3

"What Awaits Us?"

After midnight when the train
Rattles our bed,
Everything
Seems strange,
Too distant to be real.

I startle,
Still alone
With this darkness.
How can a man outlive
The midnight of a marriage?

Moon tides move souls
Close but fog may form
To outlast any love.
I have roamed each
Room while you sleep.

It is I who has not yet known you.
A full moon filters pink
Though the fog. My
Emptiness should
Always be such a soft hue.

The Things That You Were

I wander pensively
In your garden, leaving
The hospital where you died.

Here beside your roses
And deer statues
You are alive.

I feel your character
Growing in a pot
Of chicken-n-hen cactus.

The blades on your windmill
Are silent now but I know
You are here.

I look lovingly at
The oft-worn straw hat
And feel you pulsating me.

Remembered things
Weave your spirit
Square-knotted to mine.

I smile, cradling memories.
So familiar and strong
Is your presence.

For months hence
I will startle when I feel
You in the things that you were.

I round the curve beyond
The graveyard where you rest
And startle seeing a red pick-up.

Instantly the truck bed
Is packed with living
Snapshots of you.

You ride beside me
In the passenger seat
—An unwelcome hitchhiker.

When will I see,
Without seeing you
My love?

Bonnie Raingruber, "The Things That You Were," Palliative and Supportive Care, vol. 6, no. 1, pp. 89.

Lacunae

I look into your eyes, I try to talk
To touch your thoughts, your heart.
There is only emptiness I cannot reach.
Your chocolate eyes stare into the void.
Your face alien, a mask to me.
Where have you gone?
We used to talk for hours into the night.
Specificity, detail, passion
Have fled seeking oxygen elsewhere.
What do you hear when I chatter?
Do you know me? Do you see me?
There is only vacant, empty space
Where once we were one.
Necrotic love has us now.

Leaving Things Tidy

I sat in the French Provincial
Chair labeled "Alvin"
Allocated early
For her youngest son.

Today, three weeks before
Death she held court,
Cloistered in the bottom wing
Of her two-story flat, in a house

Within a house where her world
Was now. We spoke of breathing
In and out with death;
Of arrival points in life

like the day belongings
Don't matter anymore;
Of titrating worry
Within 5 ccs of functional,

And accepting so many non-options;
Of trying in the world that is
—Because nothing else works—
Of feeling illness cancel comebacks.

Referred pain, a promise from days past,
Spoke a philosophy of staying into everything;
Of keeping a calendar full to the future;
Of being a shell collector

. . . Collecting interests
And treasures in life for hobby,
Remembrances of tidier times
When living was likely.

Bonnie Raingruber, "Leaving Things Tidy," Palliative and Supportive Care, vol. 4, no. 4, pp. 429.

The Pause Between

Clouds reshape themselves
Ever so subtly.
One hardly notices
Darkness and daybreak
Twinkling in descent.
You lie recumbent
Arms folded pristine
Over chest after
Mahogany and marble
Have lost all meaning.
The pause between breaths
Sifts o'er your heart.
Silence sinks to toes.
Worry wanders away,
Drifting to sleep.
Sleep eventuates
To death.
In the silence
A cat-eyed intuition
Sees even at night
Hearing all,
Filling your lungs
With nothing but peace.
It is in the quiet
Before winter's gale
That enveloping love
Holds you safe
In tears and in joy.

Unheeded Intuitions

Tree veins sit exposed
Like arteries above ground.
Heaven can, from time to time, be seen.
Still man does not step lightly.
Rattlesnake grass
Whispers a warning.
Dead tree bones
Blanch white with age.
Perfidious, beauty hides
In a purple thistle-star.
Yellow canary seeks
Venom nectar.
Out of nowhere Alzheimer's
Rears up, showing stinger.
Elders chide and shout.
My youth did not hear.
Again I am. Again, I must
Cloak spirit with flesh.
Sounds at the ocean are eternal.

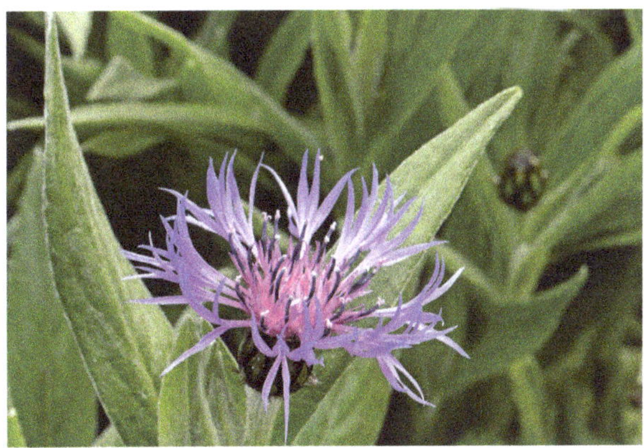

IMG 2.4

War in a Winter Tempo

Icicle claws and a caesura
Sat silent, sat breathless.
Rain and fog fought.
Fog lay too thick to sustain itself.
Rain sat ready, waiting.
Drops nearly coalesced,
Seeking the perfect
Sphere, needing enough
Internal force to form.
Icicle claws and a caesura
Sat silent, sat breathless.
Muse memory and nebula knowing
Fought. Befogged—dementia follows
You everywhere—laying
Too thick, sustaining itself.
Recollections coalesce, condensing
Into a self, seeking the perfect time,
Needing enough internal force to form.
Silently, fog punctuates itself.
In the rain and tears, rustling leaves
long since dead are finally heard.
Unseen forces on the wind take us all.
Veiled protections pile up—ready to be burnt.
Evaporating will they be cinder or smoke?
Oblivion before it coalesces
Will blind you. Like a leaf let go,
Pain fades only after it has been felt.

Canyon de Chelly

Moonbeam casts leaf shadows.
Silence works its spell.
Each raven cry is heard
Echoing like intuition.
On a ledge above the void
South of the sun, pueblo appears.
All rooms of equal size, blackened by fire, soot
Guarded by a single sentinel.
Anasazi art—triangle body, vestigial limb
Black, white, bold.
Portal of intercession
Anthropomorph with twin hair knots
Arms raised—tying Man, God.
Blood handprints
Mark each granite passing.
One rabbit fur blanket
Cradle from the cold remains.
Comfort is short, soft.
Lives knot together
Woven tight as human hair belt.
Subterranean memories spill into one plunge pool
We are as we think,
As we feel,
As we experience,
Only as long as we believe and know.

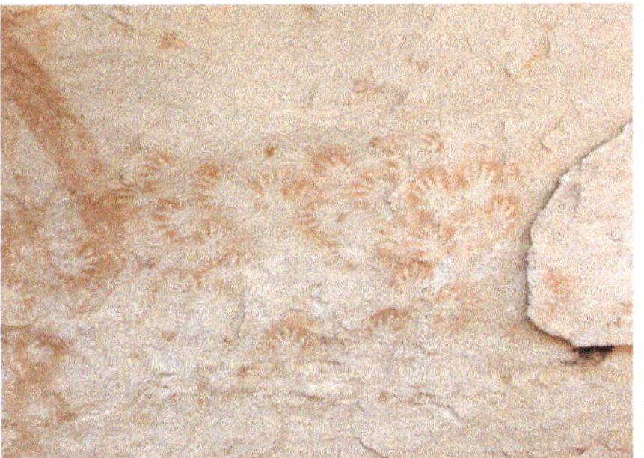
IMG 2.5

Winter in California

Ballerina jumps, raindrop bends
Landing light
Floating atop a snow
Pond at Big Trees National Park.
Snow falls sudden
From Redwood perch
Glimmering gold
With the sun.
Hidden inside a piercing wind
Alzheimer's comes—a sudden
Burning lack of belief—bringing
Us the chance to see anew.
Tinsel sound rattles
The silence, the soul.
For 500 years these redwoods
Have held peace soft inside one bosom.
Man feeds.
Photosynthesis dances
And burns the sky
Like lava.
Xylem and phloem
Circle and sing. Soubresants,
And pirouettes curtsey to joy,
Bending reverent to listen, to hear.

Spiders in the Rain

Where do spiders go in the rain?
Treacherous creatures, tender web
Hung on a tree branch with shimmered thread.
They tempt me to hose them away.

Where do the homeless go in the rain?
An urban doorway, a park bench till early dawn?
Dirt and danger are seen as I am
Looking past and through you.

Where do stray cats go in the rain?
A cold eave, a low-slung bush?
How does one find
A home after being left?

It is hard to connect
When forsaken is woven to one's DNA.
Seven generations of pain
Cry out before we are, any of us, free.

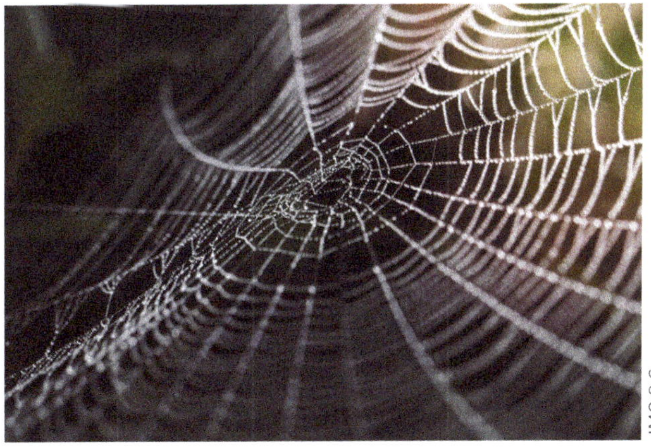

IMG 2.6

Orphan Angry

I am orphaned
Parented only by nature's magic
And angels of the earth.
Why was I left alone?
Why did Alzheimer's kidnap my mate?
Lonely echoes reverberate.
I am left to cook, clean, comfort.
We used to play every day together.
I did not ask to be a waif
Raising us both by myself.

Memories

My brain is a jar of molasses
Melting in the summer sun,
Sticking one brain cell,
Gluing it to another,
Clumping thoughts together
Like a popcorn ball
Ready to explode
And pop reality apart.

Climates

Seasons and climates
Surround each person
Each animal, each bird.
Feel who is beside you.
Who guides and nudges?
Where are you blown?
What does your essence herald?
Which is the season of your heart?

Ancestors stand behind me.
The wind envelops.
Gentle caress
We knit to tree root, to the matrix
At the heart of all.
Silence reins.
Hear as you are
Alone in the together.

Cats feel with the brush of a whisker.
Dogs know fear in an instant.
People carry a cloud with them
As cloak, sometimes as dagger.
Is the flavor of your soul
Pleasing to those who
Brush beside and into
The path which has chosen you?

A Portable Fire

You built a portable fire
Deep in the Shasta Woods
Under the rain-dripped boughs
Of a pine tree on my stormiest day.
Since then, you have remained
As a portable fire in my heart
Which almost warms
Up to satisfaction
My smoke-filled memory
So much so that I still take you
With me wherever I go.

I Thought of You Today

Memory is a corn stalk
Golden, whipped by the wind,
Delicate then gone.
Remembered times
Dust gently like pollen
Through and into me.
We are what we recall.
We are what we celebrate.

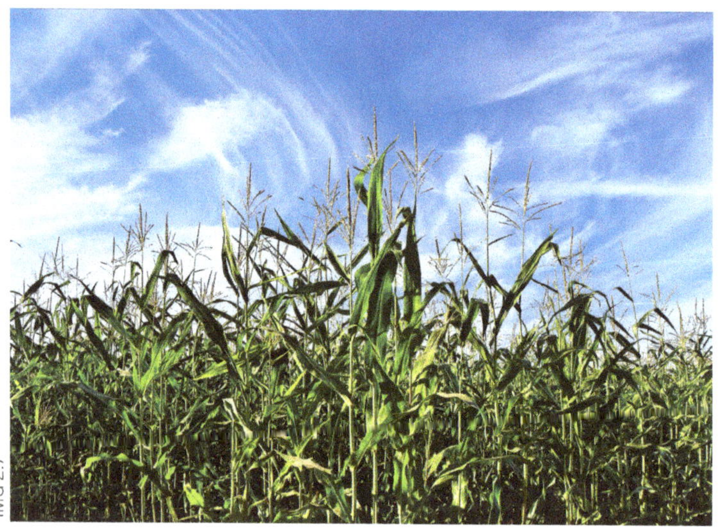

IMG 2.7

An Old Memory

On my automatic message machine, I hear
An old conversation, rewound
And played back in my mind's eye
Spliced with memory traces.
My mind travels back into our
History and word creates reality
Vivid as can be.

Your voice glides
Pulling each separate
Strand braiding my long hair,
Stroking my heartstrings,
Reverberating in stereo, hundreds
Of vintage memories tucked away in my
Picture album heart, remaining as real as today.

The Washday Find

I empty your pockets on washday to find
A half-opened piece of gum sticking to all.
Two spiral-bound notebooks full to overflowing with half written poems,
Ideas for a novel, three verses of a County-Western song
All bent beyond recognition from being smashed
By a fat wallet—a wallet full of receipts, store coupons, small bills
In disarray, tattered like a thought
That has circled your mind one too many times.
A pen leaking ink staining all—the favorite possession
Of a man who lives inside his head hearing words that must be written.
A comb missing tooth, no longer able to straighten thoughts.
Disarray—she is the mother of my husband's creativity.
He is uncensored chaos theory held inside a pair of size 36 blue Levi's
With a mind that blows with the wind to beauty, to inspiration.
In his pockets I have found why I married the man.

Drop the Leaf

A rain shower of leaves fall—
Flutters and murmurations blowing as one—
Waves of golden parchment.
In my diary I engrave a list of daily wrongs.
When will I drop these pains?
Nature sheds her flaws every November.
She knows yielding, bending humility
Is the source of power.
I listen, learning that strength
Attends a dormancy of pride.
My heart bends a knee.
Spring awaits God's tempo and timing.

A Hard-Luck Life

I lived a hard-luck life that I never owned
Posturing proud, pulling ahead.
Scars checkerboard my future
Deliberate like a chess game.
Criss-crossed cuts confine me.
Imprisoned by past pain,
Old wounds fight today's battles for me.
A scream is living inside, asking to be free.
I am making social conversation with death.
Saying hello in futile expectation
Of going home finally.

Fortunes Told

Read my palm.
Lines etched there
Nerve ending portals
Leading to a road's end.
Read my face.
See my character
Tattooed there.
Touch my spine, feel
Soul-ganglia, chakras.
See my eyes look up,
Wide-eyed like pleading silence
—Open as hope ready to explode—
God's finger bears record
And gives to man a book
Called remembrance
Written not on paper
But written in flesh.
My body is a sieve, sifting truth.
My body grows accustomed
To the pace daily life draws.
We all resemble our traits.
We become our actions in body.
Soft like a kitten
Batting the air, claw retracted.

In Your Presence

Two auras overlap us.
Your skin knows me,
Embryologically, it unfolds,
Recognizing the betweens
That live us. Differentiated,
I dance fetal-fisted,
Older than the ages.
I hear you thinking me real.
Mechanically I am turning
—A bird jerking its head
Clicking by degrees to another perspective.
Mystery is hard to manipulate.
Childlike I sparkle in your eyes.
Peace cords to my navel.
Your strength envelops me.
Your quiet pride soothes my heart.
I am whole.

Lightening Fears

Cloud to ground, earthquake lights
And stick figures dance under our Cedar.
I see you there 20 months after you passed.
Spider web memories hold my heart.
I miss you so.
Each shadow casts and reels in
Strings binding our love.
In a flash you appear.
I startle. Flashbacks
Grab my hand. Sadness
Walks with my heart.

The Path of Totality

I hold to a thin ribboned memory.
Moon shadow, the path of totality
Where Moon eclipses Sun.
Corona rings my heart to you.
Brief, too brief but those
4 minutes can burn you blind.
Protect your eyes
Remember our life
With rose colored glasses.
Reality was too hard.
Mother moon alone cradles dark, soft
Paths back to a two-person universe.

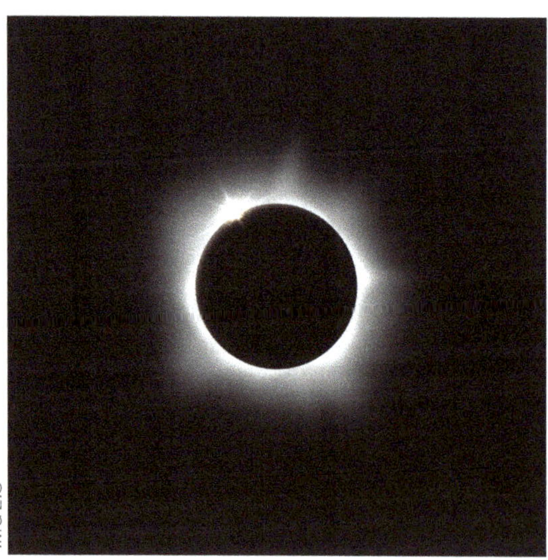

IMG 2.8

Waves of Tomorrow

Gentle breeze—
Waves to the shore
Moiré taffeta
Regular patterned, predictable.
A soft lullaby of cottonwood
Sung sweetly.
Red dawn—
Waves to the shore
Unseen tidal wave
Sudden rent.
A shriek of pain
Piercing heart.
How deep must change go?
Shorelines are carved each day.
Erosive forces have your hand.
Where do you walk?
Rounding corner, what awaits?
Waves buffet, salt tears carve another dawn.

Sunset Sifting

When our sun sets,
Night's hand bruises
Green tree to yellow gold.
Then feelings and colors
Transmute like hurt
Healing from the inside out.
Light is a golden-haired phoenix
Mouthing the gorge
Where sunlight sits last,
Pink blinking its border.

Gray zigzags black,
Lizard-like moving into
Night. Skin wrinkles,
Scurrying to let go, to get
Away from sun-bright souls.
Heat hides inside
Rocks cracking them to yawns
Showing pith, marrow,
Tonsil—heralding a son orb
Center, now returned.

Green-gone-black
Silhouettes tree soft sink,
Feather folded into evening.
Eminence is inward.
Understanding's green gold
Sits bent-bow quiet, ready
To pierce the daylight,
Logic clothing Adam's rib
With an arrowhead
Certainty sharp.

Lullaby sounds age,
And cricket songs sing melody.
Life streams converge, finding focal point
Calling it contentment. Sustenance is
Given and found, flowing soft
O'er granite rocks holding father time's
Potency. Psyche is lymph draining,
Blanketed by night's black velvet.
Our bedrock is solitude
Worn by a darkness called dream.

Rocks layer round,
Tree rings count our age
Like dermis scaled deep,
Antiquity's years, numbering pain
Are counted as comprehension.
Dexterity is rendered up. Curving brain
Bends and loosely associated shale
Are sifting darker through the sieve
Separating day and eve, precipitating
To metastasis for seven sages.

Jackson Highway

A shadow self on the ground does fall,
Circling Black Oak, reflecting there.
Dreamlands shade and reflect reality—
One dimension of that which
Creates the outline of what will be.
I am prisoner of a large patterned life,
Dark and karma-cast.
Hawk wings follow what is too fast to outrun.
A squirrel feels the cold shutter of a winged silhouette.
Come meet me tonight in dream.
Let us find our pattern on this earth
And visit at the edge of another.
There the mountain casts cold and dark,
Eclipsing spring from bits of this wintered world.

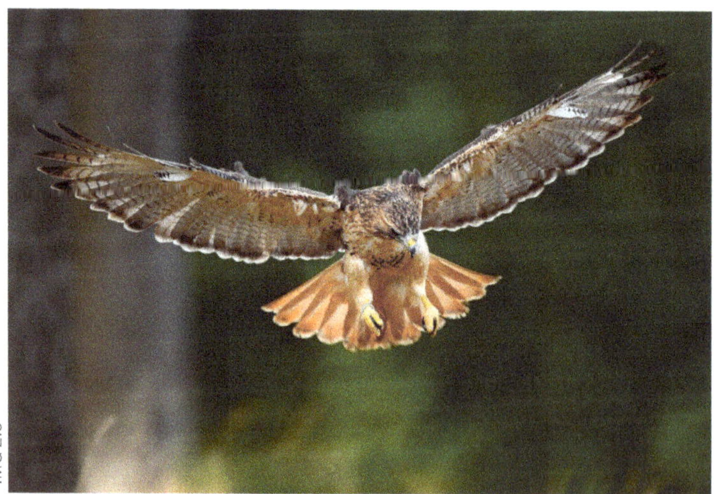
IMG 2.9

Crane Dances

Winds of the One
Blow ego prostrate.
Thigh muscles quiver and shake.
Taut, fearful—
Xylem and Phloem
Do not move in winter.
Birds smile a symphony
Ushering in spring in Bethesda,
Breathing out black
Sighing, "Ah Shaw Ne Daw."
Qi flows from the heavens
Through flaccid muscle
Healing within, healing without.
Through the five scared mountains
We pass lifetimes. From the
Palace of Eternal Frost
O'er the Golden Gate of the East
We journey together.

Cypress Forests

Gall rancors, rounding in on itself.
Woman left is callused hard.
Balloon beads string together
And amplify wrong for all to see.
Tumor trees swell to safety
Bitten by insect bitter.
Bandages always show.
White flags are held high,
Defying each heart surrender.
Fear is rheumatic armor,
Amplifying uneven,
Lonely, gnarled, dark
At the edge of the ocean.

Dream Carcass

Such a strong backbone
To lie naked
What was once fish
Now flanked by tail
And a red-eyed head.
Feathery without flesh
Nothing remains
But hairlike bone.

Such a strong dream
To lie naked
What was once my future
Now flanked by failure
And a red-eyed hurt
Feathery without flesh
Nothing remains
Nothing . . .

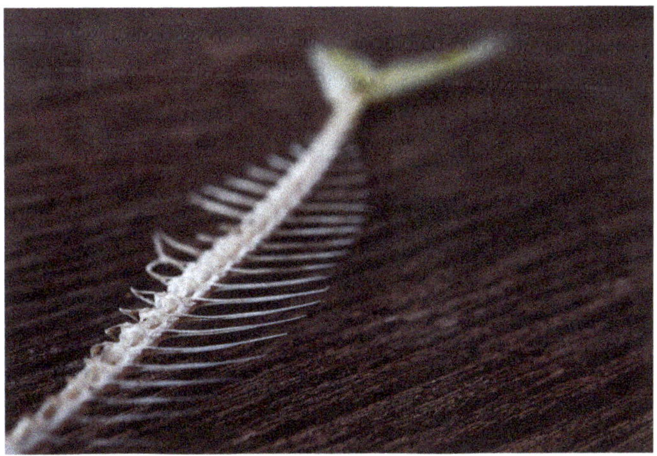

IMG 2.10

Bonnie Raingruber, "Dream Carcass," Palliative and Supportive Care, vol. 4, no. 4, pp. 431.

Changes

Red breaks through green,
Birthing two tulips.

Stop o'ertakes go.
Relationships bloom and pause.

Fast-forwarded to gone, it takes
Two clicks to do things differently.

Chocolate-dipped cones collapse within
When the ice cream has melted away.

The tide filters past,
Settling sand 1/8 of an inch out

From under any certainty
My footprints have known.

Celebrate—change is from the cradle.
Growth is a tender bud.

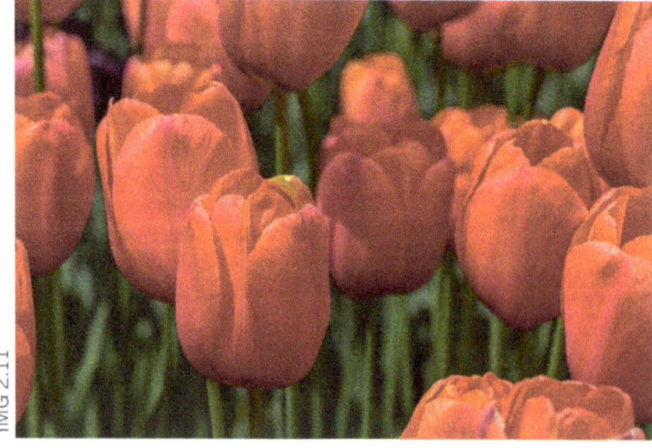

IMG 2.11

Weeping Wall

Kai-ne-sava, ash spirit,
Cloaked in turkey-feather, rabbit skin
Lied then took my life.

I was burnt orange with pain.
Anger spiraled with DNA, etching dark.
Past-present-eternity merged.

Navel Kiva connected heaven-earth
Painting recombinant history on stone spire.
Teal layers, blood handprint on rock.

Ancestor faces guarded earth-mother.
Virgin River flowed 300 to 1300 AD,
Then disappeared like dinosaur womb.

Droplets still seep heavy into stone
Percolating without end. Worn down
But not forgotten, circling again.

Metate breathes, grinding Karma.
Corn crop cycles live on
Past the time of the changing.

Collecting 1,500 years
Water swells to hurt in limestone breast.
Rain tears hit solid granite.

Lightning cracks creation and finds a way.
Champagne bubbles ripple effervescent
Bleeding out and over mountain falls.

Deep energy evaporates.
Zion is release within.
Anasazi, my ancient enemy, walk with me

Back to the place of the beginning.
Let go with the wind. Find High Spruce Pueblo
Protection, absent ladder to the past.

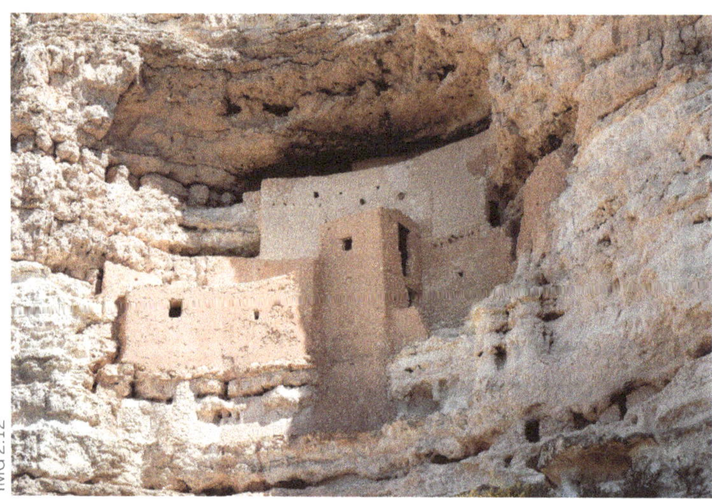
IMG 2.12

Into Tuition

Sitting with pregnant belly
Late at night, held
Soft inside rocking chair.
Swaying in rhythm
Knowing and comfort
Square knot together.

Sunlight mirrors
Gold on Zion Park
Curvilinear like the fold
Of ancient angel wing
Insight flashes
Then retracts.

Tension and release. Bow is bent
Then shot. Action is without effort.
Breathing in, breathing out.
Motor stone rubs ground corn.
Hopi mother grinds circles into tomorrow,
Feeling the pulse of life, internal.

Pulled by the past,
Drawn by hope.
We are all shaped
By our intent. Lightning
Quick, then gone,
In coincidence we finally see.

Each life ties to another.
We know all is and needed to be.
Good and bad disappear.
Judgment does not know.
We evolve anew.
Thought lives to grow the future.

Gaelic Gardens

Weeds whisker earth.
Black walnut trees graft
English forefather
History's veins
Abandon ancestor tree.
Impression is a footprint
Every generation follows.
Madrones shed their past,
Curling soft to sun.
Every flower finds its own place.
Forests molt. Clear-cut habits
Shed us clean like lizard tails
Left in a trap. Each genre must
Be born with the sun to survive.
From thicket-curse
Slight rises up,
Karmic in her reach.
We all shall be again.
Hold your darkness.
Hold your silence. Hear.

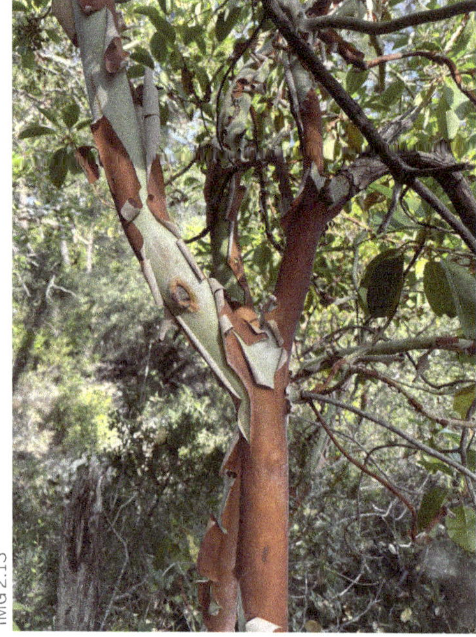

IMG 2.13

Teotihuacan

Mexican city of the Gods
Abandoned by its own, tradition was torn
And temples blazoned 1,000 years hence.
Today gargoyles only, watch ethics
Guarding what cannot be left.

Storm Gods took the city.
Curved-lip fangs smiled deception.
Flattened mustache stones silenced life's breath.
Human sacrifice hurls its pain open-mouthed,
Statuing strong to rupture virgin dispensations.

Larger than life, darkness will dance.
When will feathered serpents build
Softness as protection and shed the scale?
Tree roots are hands one season extends, grasping mother
Earth. We are watered by reptile genomes and the flow.

Our plain exterior hosts elaborate selves.
The unexpected lives pregnant inside
Every frame. Puzzle-piece meaning will again
Greco conversation in the town square. Each mouth
Speech scrolls, perpetuating idea anon.

In an age when placidity would not
Sit still with itself, wrinkled stone skin,
Cracked gray, letting wealth adhere like wisdom.
And hunchbacked man became vessel to knowledge,
Cradling an adaptation, now extinct.

In Teotihuacan, each apartment courtyarded
Its shrine. Rituals structured the day.
Action figures postured movement.
One race ventured out supreme.
Decaying teeth collared dark-jeweled agency.

Calendar bowls outlive their usefulness.
Anaerobic orange turns hornstone black. A civilization
Without metal is axed out by obsidian. Masks only
Warm the face of past dead. And in the chill
Night ushers over progress, Aztecs overtake us, still.

Double Exposure

God looks down and is confused.
He tries to follow the zigzag pattern,
My rickrack path.

But he cannot
For there is no focus,
No focus for my soul.

There are only double exposures, disjointed images
Appearing superimposed, one-on-another
Abruptly fading out, starting up somewhere else.

My path is a checkerboard pinwheel,
Whirling and fanning out in all directions,
Following each potential, never reaching conclusion.

My life is a disjointed picture
Pandemonium leading everywhere,
Having many textures and complexities.

I am an oil-splattered painting by a master
With the focal point
Strung across cold canvas.

The Dragon of Nothingness

Shadow is eyelid to earth.
Curtains are drawn each eve.
Psyche can take in only so much.
Passion waits upon the midnight solstice.
A sigh stretches and prepares the way.

Leaves brown before they go,
And then umbrella-out to summer shade.
An eagle wings with the wind, gliding before
She takes to flight. Ego can only carry
So much. Awareness must cloud to safety.

I cannot see too stark a reality.
Rapid stirrings keep a bark basket
From burning. Denial shields
Calm in my heart. Sunset prisms
Pull inward, shading gray.

Focus settles into itself. Civilization
Is pulsed by what it takes in—
And yet this decade trips over itself,
Rushing, stuttering ahead—bereft of sleep.
It will not stop; it will not know.

By contrast we are born. Cycles
Define us. Sunlight shows itself
In seasons. An eye shaded is able
To see. Shadows foretell what was.
They glimmer truth rivulets.

Night, the dragon of nothingness.
Burns and breathes life. She is protector,
Progenitor of who we will be.
Come dance in darkness. Come sing
A song of shadow, come herald in the day.

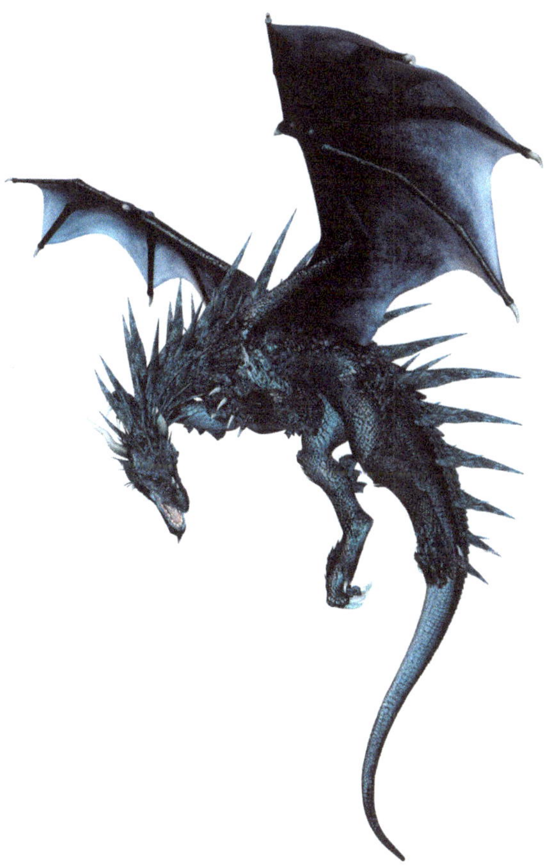

IMG 2.14

Apple Pancakes

It was the time of Apple Pancakes.
Those are the days I miss the most.
Every Saturday we went out for breakfast.
I sat close to you in the booth
Savoring thin sliced Gravensteins
Held in our pancakes—an old German recipe,
A family together in a family run restaurant.
Why didn't I realize those days would die,
You would die and I would sit alone
Missing the time of Apple Pancakes?
I still desire those days years after
The restaurant closed and the town moved on
Without reserving a happy place, any place for me.

Dropped Connection

I can't hear the sound of your voice anymore.
Deep, grounded, strong.
I can't call. I want to.
Sounds would echo into
Chambers of my heart
Valves open, blood flowing, feeling alive.
Your voice was lighthouse
Bringing poems, books, hopes
To guide me safely home.
Yet I know your voice is sound only
Without touch, without smile.
Like the wind passing
Going away from and beyond me.
I would grab hold if I could.
My fingers try to squeeze empty space.
But air, sound, life currents
Can't be held
They flow to
Another fate
Another mate.

Everywhere

Whack-a-mole
Memories of you appear
As I drive to the grocery store.
You are everywhere we visited.
—On Bianchi Lane where we bought
That roll top desk for our house,
At the church where we played chess,
On the American river
Where we first held hands.
Your thumb fit mine perfectly.

Weekday rituals: breakfast,
Dinnertime, sitting at the river
Gone. Like meaning broken
—A wine glass shattered,
An accident I could not stop.
One soul is missing
From my universe yet
A galaxy sits empty
Uninhabited, without definition,
Without structure, backbone.

I saw myself through your eyes.
Now there is no reflection in the mirror.
If I remember enough
Will you come back?
Can we start anew?
I want to be the woman I was
On our wedding day.
In memory, I am 30 years younger
Made fresh by your
Acquaintance, your love.

You were my nexus.
Each thought and action, each day
Led to you and yours.
You still pop into memory
Two years after your death.
You appear and reappear
In my heart and mind.
I revisit each place we went
In remembrance, in tribute to you.
How I miss you, my love.

Eroded and Away

Swimming in the wind, I am
Buffeted here, there, every which way.
Tree roots claw earth, trying to ground.
Erosion has left them exposed, alone, dry.
Since your passing protection
Has blown and is gone.

Spanish moss holds to branch
For life and in death. Wind whipped worry
Whiplashes between real and tragic.
Hidden pain herniates.
The past explodes. Birds litter a field
Looking like old carpet.

As the wind pulls the grass
Up and out by its roots
Tree bone branches break
—Corpses still hang on trunk noose.
Lives that were splinted together
Try to heal, try to heal.

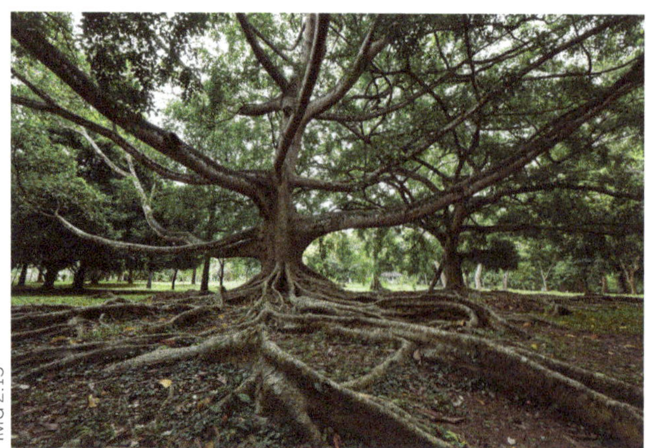
IMG 2.15

Chinese Pistachio Trees

It is the time of the Chinese Pistachio
Blazing red, golden, yet green.
Your passion fancied the red.
But this year I am left alone.
Sad rains over me.
We loved this season of life
Together last year.
Will you still
Reach for my hand
Each fall, softly with the silence
Of a fallen leaf?
Know I can hear you
In my heart.

What shadow self remains on earth
After funeral tears are bone dry?

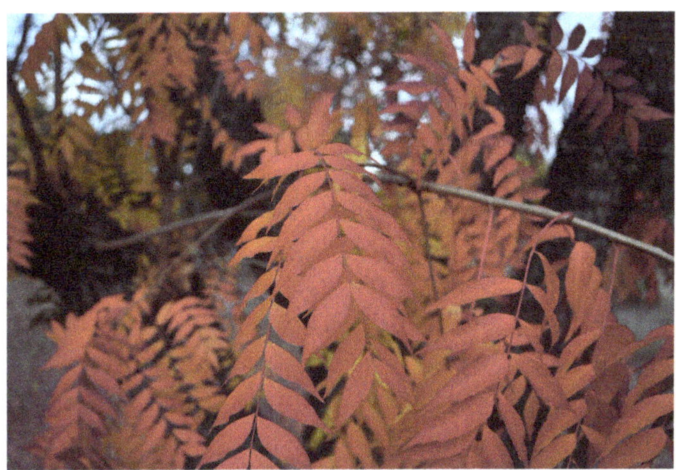

IMG 2.16

Denial

Bull frogs don't sleep.
Snakes see with their eyes closed.
Transparent eyelids are protection drawn.
Denial works too. Close the shade.
Alzheimer's is too much to look at straight on.
You must invite friends to visit
To tell you what you don't want to know.

Even caterpillars use
All 4,000 muscles
To crawl away from bad news.
Don't listen to carefully
That whistling in the woods might be
A mountain lion hunting in the dark.
Tigers can't taste, but they will eat you at night.

Dragon flies can't walk,
Their legs are for landing and taking off only
To escape pain quickly.
Guinea pigs are herd animals,
They require one another.
Switzerland makes you buy two.
Alone won't do.

Octopuses regularly turn
Off their brain
To think with their tenacles.
We all need to avoid overload.
Brains short circuit with too much bad news.
Just ask the catfish cousin, electrophorus
—760 volts of sadness per shock zaps you silly.

Turn your head upside down.
Drink in comfort food.
Be a filter feeder Flamingo.
God knew creation should
Not see the world straight up.
That's why cheetahs can't roar.
If you purr at a threat, it settles into oblivion.

Butterflies

I have to sit still
Absolutely still,
Not to flutter away.

See the human pointing
—Noticing I have stopped
Midair as hummingbird.

My worried wing
Beats so fast, heart
Cannot keep up.

I am stuck in
Not changing.
Frozen by fear.

O'errun by possibilities
Flying all at once in
My face, flying so fast.

I am a catatonic statue, paused
Waxy and electric with rage.
Can you hear the static

My head holds? I have
Settled into one corner
Calm enough to control.

I am a white winged demon,
Or a monarch on flower thrown,
Flitting and racing from this

Thought to its tangent,
Tangled and knotted--darting
And wringing anxiety dry.

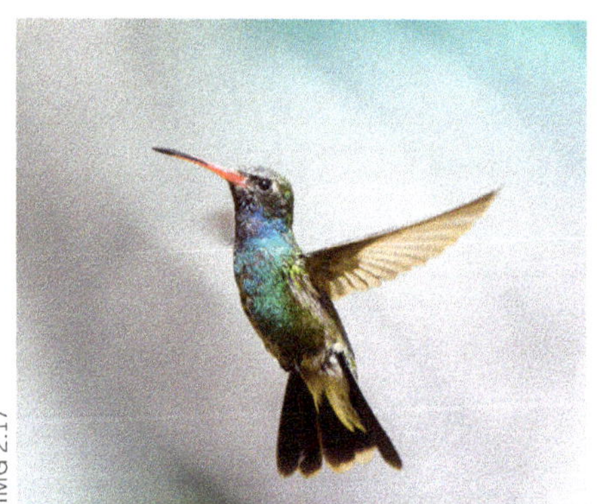
IMG 2.17

Spiraling the Drain

Water runs counterclockwise
Down the drain in Australia
Pulled by tractor beams.
Love and loss are energy vortexes
Quicksand tornados
Taffy stretched and sticky
Spiraling, circling, solidifying tomorrow.
I resist the inertia of your OHM.
Centrifugal force has me.
I try to step straight line forward
Yet I am tetherball laced to your life
Traveling around memories of our connection
Seeking center, seeking self, seeking you.

Blind Pretense

It has been one of those
Life-is-a-bore
Tangle-haired days
Where transparency
Tones are heard in the way
You are and everyone
Plus their dog can see
Motivation has freeze-dried
Cement sore inside your mouth
Tasteless and bland
As conveyor-belted routine
So that you just don't care
Who sees into your soul
While you pretend
No one does see
And they are as
Blind as thee.

Depression

Cemented in shale,
I am a stream in drab colors,
Clay-gray is desperation
Cow-skull crowned.

Maintaining momentum,
I am walking fast over rock moss,
Balancing before my soul slips
Wish-wasted into the stream.

Standing soaked, tired out,
I am two-toned-dyed hair,
Corn shuck showering
Down and out.

Black Widow

Spin me a web, strong
Enough to hold a hurt heart.
Like black satin, one tender thread
Spun at a time,
Love, an engram, lingers,
Tying tomorrow to a shroud.
A beginning kiss
Tastes hope before biting
The sweet death.

Mister Inspiration

You married
The artist in me forever.
And death has not divorced us.
Your contract requires
You continue on
As creativity's agent
For none other has shared
The slums of my growth.

Bring me a picture to write
In the early dawn when
Image becomes word. Take
Me on a journey to fresh worlds
That peek forth from a country
Road where scenes capture
My mind and whisper sunrise
Stories into the ear of my pen.

My eyes rejoice.
One hundred poem colors
Right themselves
As we travel through the air
Feeding country freedom.
My Self blooms when
Summertime rests softly atop my skin
And peace warms a tan line around my soul.

Pilot me along unknown roads
And help me discover what I have yet to see.
Drive me into a new perspective
And rattle calcified truth while
Cruising experience's bumpied road.
Invite a freshness-of-appreciation
To co-pilot our adventure
But never, never reveal the destination!

Ignite my imagination if you dare
And edit the tale it spawns.
I will, in turn,
Sign your name
To our creations
And put the royalty check
In the mail, posted to
Mr. Inspiration.

The Lost Sheep of Sleep

When sleep won't come . . .
To cuddle aches that are my body,
Embracing mangled mind-pain,
When eyeballs stare at the ceiling
Over blank eternity,
Caught in the spin-cycle,
Knowing-and-not
Turing around and around,
Agitating up recalcitrant,
Washing awareness clean
Of lamb-like experience,
Shaking-away serenity
Leaving a suspended animation
Wakefulness which won't let
The muscles holding my reality
Relax and let-go-of this fried-eyed, state of mind
Holding my eyelashes up
Ninety-nine minutes after sleeping pills
Dissolve and images dance
Trying-to-quiet sound collages
Conflicted-in-my mind,
Those loud-mouthed voices,
Who possess a fungus infested
Focus, who need to empty
The filing cabinet attention is
Into a forever-never land
Like compulsive computer
Downloading, before I doze.

Sitting at My Desk Lost

Have you ever looked up driving a road
You have known for 10 years
Suddenly not knowing where you are?
Have you ever wondered what's like
To not know how to get home?
That's always the first question with Alzheimer's.
Have you ever looked up from your busy life
And asked "how did I get here?"
On a day like every other day
Has everything suddenly felt foreign?
What is it about confusion, clarity & the familiar
That helps us see what is,
Where we are, & how to get home?

Trust

Your palm,
Cat paw-stretches
Itself firm to my thigh.

We are traveling
Home this Christmas Eve
Night has been blanket to our love.

In the dark we have shown ourselves.
The most primitive reflexes only
Happen when we rely on another.

From the crib a first reflex
Repeats itself. The familiar brings
Comfort, budding growth.

Wicker basket strong, men
And women weave shared time
Together, one strand at a time.

You must relax into love,
And always believe
It will hold.

Kit Carson Trail

Trees meld into shared trunks in the high country.
That brings stability, that brings warmth.
Merging like two people living a 30-year marriage.
Snow and lightning strike Elephant-back peak.
A shard of pain snaps branched joy
Leaving widow twig—a tree half alive, half dead.
Listening for the sound of snow falling
Liquid tears, a waterfall softly singing
Calling, echoing like a lost mate.
White ghost trees—bark stripped bare
Stand without life, marking the way.
A patch of pink wildflowers
Lost in a world of wild
Never noted on the outbound trail
Are seen heading home.
Insight dances only in the sunlight
Like a monarch butterfly migrating home.
But when the bird songs stop
A mate is out of territory.
Bees taste every fireweed blossom
Before moving to a new flower, a new relationship.
"Ours" is a small world until it is no longer
Then it becomes gigantic grey gorge.
Death took the part of me that is missing.
Lonely is a flavor, bitter, cold, burnt.
Waiting for Spring's wild bloom.

Bright Dancer

Evening's light mottled a path.
Twin shadows led our way.
Our hips held hands, walking
Us along the American River.

My lifeline enveloped the fleshy
Fold of your thumb.
Mistletoe bouquets
Bridled the night air fresh.

We pierced the river
Pretty with such insight as shines
Relationships new, feeling flexible as cats
Doing Yoga on the windowsill, toe-fanning free.

A soft smile lipped up from the little
Boy inside your hurt and together
We whistled innocent
Ice-cream truck melodies.

Quiet coalesced
To curd out a rhyme,
Singing us centered as peaches
Warmed by the summer sun.

Ultimately it is the process
Not the prize,
Not the red rose you bring,
That a woman weeps for.

It is in being
Women hear
Certainty's sound,
Hair-chested and solid.

The ovum hope descends,
Ripens love. Heart-held power
Flows wispy; wearing
White gossamer, it trails gently.

You must lap at love,
Savoring the sip,
For lovers return to mind,
One smile at a time.

Precept upon precept
Night golden, we grow.
Subtle is the spirit
Whispering truth.

A we focus unfurls
Playful as a mistress, outside
Obligation's circle: all the while
A me focus faints fast away.

You sing my heart high, Bright Dancer.
Together we ripped February from the calendar,
And still I hear your footsteps
Pattering expectant past my pride.

But tell me, do you
Count the seasons
That we mark together
The same as I?

Credits

IMG 2.1: Copyright © 2012 Depositphotos/dndavis.
IMG 2.2: Copyright © 2018 Depositphotos/martinsvanags.
IMG 2.3: Copyright © 2015 Depositphotos/Elnur_.
IMG 2.4: Copyright © 2021 Depositphotos/frederiquewacquier.
IMG 2.5: Copyright © 2011 Depositphotos/PiLens.
IMG 2.6: Copyright © 2023 Depositphotos/laurenthive.
IMG 2.7: Copyright © 2013 Depositphotos/kotafoty.
IMG 2.8: Copyright © 2013 Depositphotos/Elymas.
IMG 2.9: Copyright © 2016 Depositphotos/OndrejProsicky.
IMG 2.10: Copyright © 2016 Depositphotos/antpkr.
IMG 2.11: Copyright © 2023 Depositphotos/Posonsky.
IMG 2.12: Copyright © 2024 Depositphotos/MarkCastiglia.
IMG 2.13: Copyright © 2022 Depositphotos/majzengelter.gmail.com.
IMG 2.14: Copyright © 2021 Depositphotos/PantherMediaSeller.
IMG 2.15: Copyright © 2010 Depositphotos/DmitryRukhlenko.
IMG 2.16: The Fun Chronicles, https://www.flickr.com/photos/196406308@N04/53334539305/in/photolist-8oxfQd-8UkbeN-8Uh8JP-8Uhf2H-2kV9ACY-5NEFkT-9BStxj-2iP7eB3-2iP9WPN-gG6rqy-gG6T3B-8eEtuu-2pfYigh-2pfYU56-8eBaQM-8eEvj7-2pfZsov-2pfSAN2-9BSjFn-2n9KPnB-2n9KPrK-2n9TWic-2n9Repk-2n9Re7S-2n9TWuK-2pfZsB6-2pfYRKG-2pfYRQM-2pfYRHx-2pfYRKm-2pfYihV, 2023.
IMG 2.17: Copyright © 2017 Depositphotos/glassandnature.

Writing as a Reflective Practice

A main purpose of writing and all reflective practice activities is to let go of images and feelings that remain on your mind and in your awareness at the end of a difficult clinical day. Skill in writing develops over time with repeated practice. It is not important that you create a perfect poem. If in writing, you have let go of lingering impressions you have succeeded.

Before beginning to write it works best to settle into a contemplative mood. Some people do that by listening to music, by spending a moment in nature, by meditating, by reading others' poetry, by holding a cat, by dancing or passing a few minutes in any relaxing activity. Since everyone is different, it is worth the effort to experiment and find out what activity works best for you.

Next, focus on what it was about the day that remains in your awareness, what you feel strongly about and can't stop pondering. Jot down short phrases; paint a picture of the main emotions, sensations, and experiences. Ask yourself what else reminds you of those same feelings. List those ideas as they may become additional stanzas of the same poem.

The introspective nature of writing is healing; it refines one's character, distills human meanings, catalogues and bears witness to poignant moments from practice. Writing about one's lived experience is healing. It allows one to see, to peer into complex situations, to become a more caring nurse. The activities in the following sections are designed to develop your writing skill and provide you a way to learn from your practice.

Enhance Your Practice Activities

Look through all the poems in this book. List an emotion that is the primary theme for the husband in each poem. Do the same for all the wife's poems. How do those emotions differ? What is similar among them?

Which poem in this book was your favorite? Please explain why you liked that poem.

Look through all the poems in this book. Select the poem that you think conveyed the strongest emotion. Have you experienced any situations or feelings similar to those described in that poem? Please explain what about that poem reminded you about something in your own experience.

Look through all the poems in this book. Select a poem that emphasizes emotions and feelings that are the most strikingly different from anything you have experienced in your life. What new insights, if any, did you gain by reflecting on the meaning of the poem? How would your emotions or actions have differed compared to those of the author?

Select one poem from this book and explain why it belongs in a collection of poetry about Alzheimer's and dementia.

Identify a poem you can imagine yourself sharing with a family member experiencing Alzheimer's or dementia. How would you introduce the poem? What would you say to convey their experience might be different or similar to that described in the poem? What would be the value of sharing such a poem? Which poem would you *not* feel comfortable sharing? Please explain your answer.

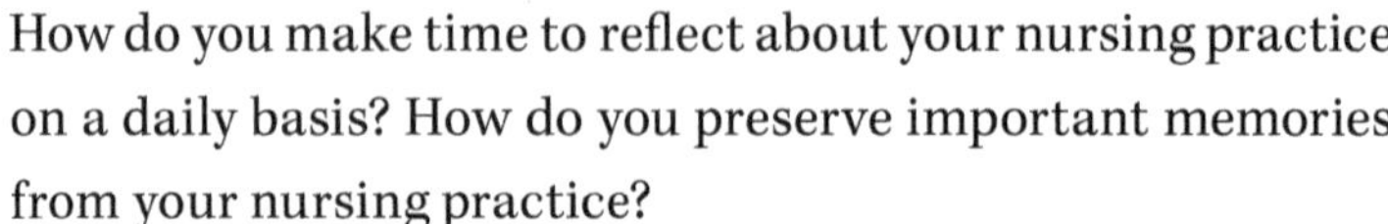

How do you make time to reflect about your nursing practice on a daily basis? How do you preserve important memories from your nursing practice?

What sort of clinical situations do you spend the most time reflecting about after the shift is over? Describe a time that reflecting about your practice was helpful to you.

What is the main theme of the poem “The Kite”? Why might someone experiencing Alzheimer’s feel that the disease was “willing the flight”? What other diseases “take control of” one’s life?

Many of the poems in this book are written about a physical place. Describe a place you have recently been that was similar to a place described in one of these poems, or write about a place you have visited that brought you a sense of comfort or peace.

Select one poem from this book and describe the beliefs and values that are woven into the poem.

Select a poem from this book that portrays the "speaker" feeling different than you do, and select a poem that portrays the "speaker" feeling something you have also felt at least once. Identify which poem portrayed something you have felt and a poem you could not relate to. Talk about those similarities and differences and what they mean.

Select a poem from this book that includes a vivid image. How was the poet affected by the image portrayed in the poem? Think back to a time from your nursing practice when a vivid image remained with you for an extended period. How did that image affect you?

Reread the poem "Coves." What do the lines "I understood the vainness of my hope to slow my seaward surge. As well as I could I savored coves I'd come to know" mean?

Select a poem from this book that teaches you something. What is it you learned? What was it in the poem that helped you learn?

What is the most important message about patient care contained in any one of these poems? Please explain your answer.

Reflective Practice Exercises: Learning to Write

Look through all the poems in this book. Select the poem that did the best job of weaving literal descriptions and metaphoric meanings together. Which lines were literal; which were an analogy?

Look through all the poems in this book and select the poem with the best ending line. What was the ending line of the poem, and why did you like it? What makes for a good ending to a poem?

Look through the poems in this book that are written in the first person. What's the title of that poem? How does writing in the first person engage the reader so they can relate to and connect with the experience described?

Look though all the poems in this book and find one that describes a place or a feeling or a person by including a lot of specific details and nuances. What is the title of that poem? How does being literal work to communicate an overall mood or make a poem understandable to others?

Take a walk around your house, around your community, or around your workplace. Notice an object or scene that holds some meaning for you. Use your imagination to take a picture of that object in your mind. Write down a concrete description of that object or scene. Then begin a list of "loose associations" and meanings associated with that object or scene. What is the first thing it reminds you of? What other objects, situations, or experiences are related in terms of having a similar

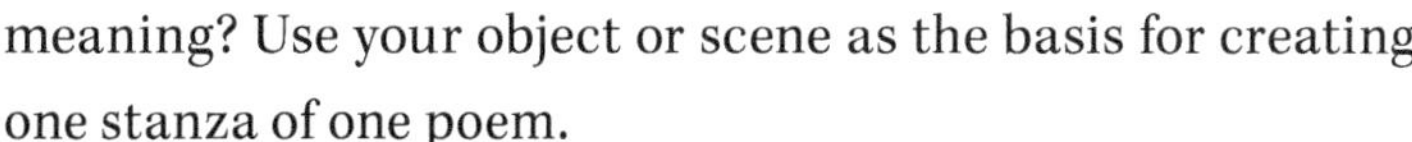

meaning? Use your object or scene as the basis for creating one stanza of one poem.

Select one poem from this book that has an interesting opening. What were the poet's concerns at the beginning of this poem? How did they change by the end of the poem?

Look through all the poems in this book for an example of the use of alliteration. Alliteration involves using words that either sound alike or begin with the same letter in close proximity in a poem. For example, "Breeze battered" and "from flake to falls" are short examples in these poems of alliteration. Describe another example that you noticed. Why is the use of alliteration in poetry effective?

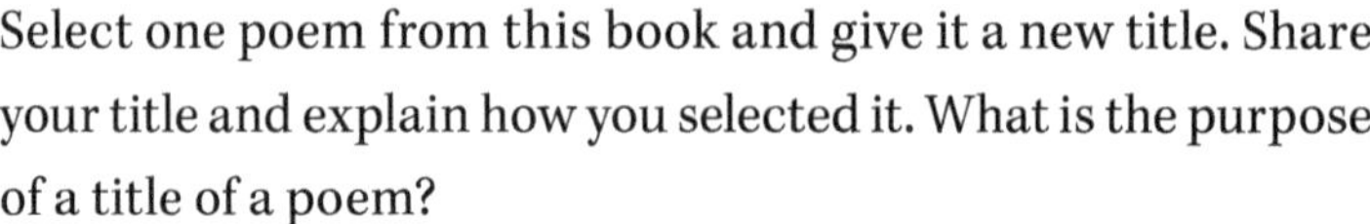

Select one poem from this book and give it a new title. Share your title and explain how you selected it. What is the purpose of a title of a poem?

What is the value of considering multiple examples of a given feeling in everyday life? Why do poets use varied references and multiple meanings in a given poem? Describe an example of this from within this collection.

Read some of the poems in this book aloud. Select the most powerful phrase from any poem in this book. Why did that phrase catch your attention? Describe why you liked or noticed the language used in that phrase.

Helpful Hints for Writing About Your Practice-Based Experience

1. Pay attention to shifts in your mood. Take note of situations that remain in your awareness. Keep a notebook or cell phone notes page handy to capture your insights.
2. Keep a journal. Write without paying attention to sentence structure, grammar, or spelling. Forget about whether your poem is good enough. Just write. Cathartic writing and telling the story is healing (Walker, 2002).
3. Reflect on your clinical experiences and select one event, impression, or memory to describe. What is it about that event, impression, or memory that was associated with the strongest feeling?
4. Reflect on the felt shifts and new ways of seeing/experiencing associated with the event, impression, or memory (Gendlin, 1962).
5. Ask yourself how this experience differs from or contrasts with others' experience? How is this event, impression, or memory connected with your own sense of the past, present, or future?
6. Focus on the unclear edges of the experience. Fill in the missing spaces in your memory with how you feel now.
7. Claim your experiences. Look for an analogy that explains how you feel. Weave a poem around the analogy so that several lines of the poem relate to the analogy and several lines relate to your literal experience. Alternate the metaphorical and literal descriptions. Use the analogy to show the reader your experience and to paint a visual picture. Meaning emerges from the free play of images and analogies in poetry.

8. Play with repetition. The repetition in poetry and in metaphors reinforces a multitude of meanings. In poetry, experience and thought merge as the message is conveyed in a "multilayered, figure-ground sort of architecture" (Akhtar, 2000, p. 235). Poetry is like Escher's paintings, only in words.
9. Use alliteration by including words that begin with the same letter or sound. Or try your hand at incorporating a rhyming scheme.
10. Juxtapose related images and meanings. Write stanza 2 about a variant example of stanza 1. Where else would you see the concept or feeling you are writing about?
11. Ask yourself "What else does this lingering feeling remind me of?" Be tangential; describe multivalent impressions.
12. Describe an actual experience, place, or feeling. Include as many details and nuances as possible. Being literal works to communicate an overall mood and to make it understandable to others.
13. Try experimenting. Make up words or use words in a new way. Use nouns as verbs. Use the thesaurus to look up new and interesting-sounding words. Edit out the "chain of OFs" if you overuse them. Try eliminating extraneous words. Ask yourself if any words can be deleted without changing the meaning of your poem.
14. Speak from the first-person point of view. Engage the reader by being clear about and introducing who the speaker is. Let your reader know who is sharing the story so that they can relate to and connect with the experience.

15. Try to use Anglo-Saxon words rather than Latin words. Such short, powerful words in phrases work well to express intense feelings. Be bold. Poetry requires a distillation and intensification of meaning (Wheelock, 1963).
16. End with a powerful, memorable, or striking phrase that is concise and to the point.

Helpful Hints for Creating a Drawing About Your Clinical Experience

1. Choose colors that match your feeling. Intense colors such as black and red, as well as deep hues, work well to express powerful emotions.
2. Use contrasting textures or colors to express your feelings. Simple is powerful and liberating!
3. Try stark images. Experiment with what they have to say.
4. Remember the point of completing a poem or a drawing is to express your feelings. There is no right or wrong way to develop a poem or a drawing. Don't worry about whether your poem or drawing is good enough. If you express how you feel or felt, you have succeeded.

References

Akhtar, S. (2000). Mental pain and the cultural ointment of poetry. *International Journal of Psychoanalysis, 81*(2), 229–243.

Bachelard, G. (1969). *The poetics of space.* Beacon Press.

Benner, P., & Wrubel, J. (1989). *The primacy of caring.* Addison-Wesley.

Connelly, J. (1999). Being in the present moment: Developing the capacity for mindfulness in medicine. *Academic Medicine, 74*(4), 420–424.

Crawford, T. H. (1993). *Modernism, medicine & William Carlos Williams.* The University of Oklahoma Press.

Dewey, J. (1910). *How we think.* D.C. Heath and Company.

Friedrich, M. J. (1999). Passion for poetry: Compassion for others. *Journal of the American Medical Association, 281*(13), 1159–1161.

Gendlin, E. T. (1962). *Experiencing and the creation of meaning.* The Free Press of Glencoe.

Holmes, B., & Gregory, D. (1998). Writing poetry: A way of knowing nursing. *Journal of Advanced Nursing, 28*(6), 1191–1194.

Kemmis, S. (1985). Action research and the politics of reflection. In D. Boud, R. Keogh, & D. Walker (Eds.), *Reflection: Turning experience into learning* (pp. 139–163). Nicholas.

Linney, B. J. (2000). Can you take your soul to work? *The Physician Executive, 26*(2), 59–62.

Loughran, J. J. (2002). Effective reflective practice: In search of meaning in learning about teaching. *Journal of Teacher Education, 53*(1), 33–43.

Schon, D. (1983). *The reflective practitioner: How professionals think in action.* Basic Books.

Walker, B. L. (2002). Stories and the brain: Making crucial connections. *Archives of Psychiatric Nursing, 16*(6), 241–242.

Wheelock, J. H. (1963). *What is poetry?* Scribner's.

Wylie, M. S., & Simon, R. (2002). Discoveries from the black box. *Psychotherapy Networker, 26*(5), 26–37.